The Clinician's Guide

to

Better Birth after Caesarean

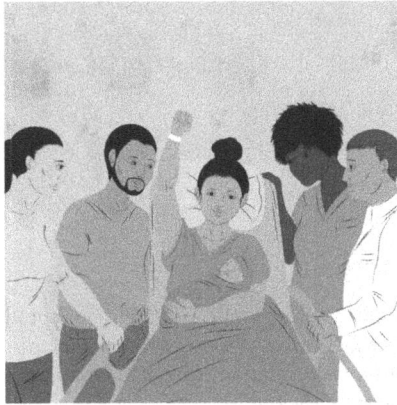

Dr. Hazel Keedle, PhD

Praeclarus Press. LLC
©2025 Hazel Keedle. All rights reserved
www.PraeclarusPress.com

Praeclarus Press, LLC
2504 Sweetgum Lane
Amarillo, Texas 79124 USA
806-367-9950

www.PraeclarusPress.com

DISCLAIMER

The information contained in this publication is advisory only and is not intended to replace sound clinical judgment or individualized patient care. The author disclaims all warranties, whether expressed or implied, including any warranty as the quality, accuracy, safety, or suitability of this information for any particular purpose.

ISBN: 978-1-946665-80-5

Cover Design: Ken Tackett
Developmental Editing: Kathleen Kendall-Tackett
Copyediting: Chris Tackett
Layout & Design: Nelly Murariu

Table of Contents

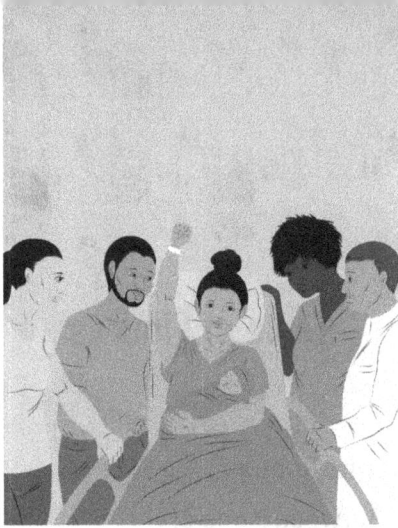

Dedication

This book is dedicated to the "Hazel" Midwifery Group Practice at the Royal Hospital for Women, Sydney, Australia.

There is no greater honour for me than having a midwifery continuity of care practice named after me and I thank you for that honour.

I dedicate this book to the "Hazel" midwives, keep up the amazing support that you provide all the women that access your MGP.

Table of Figures

Acknowledgements

I would like to thank the willing workshop participants that attended my birth after caesarean workshops and inspired me to write this, my second book. I am thankful for their willingness to share their experiences and their openness to be challenged and gain new knowledge.

Thank you to the clinicians that share their stories in this book. They are amazing midwives and doulas from Australia and Indonesia, and I appreciate their honesty and wisdom. Thank you, Dr. Kirsten Small, for adding your wisdom to this book.

I would also like to thank my friends and work colleagues who make is such a joy to work with and who share in our passion for midwifery and education.

I would like to thank my mentors, Professor Hannah Dahlen, Professor Virginia Schmied, and Associate Professor Elaine Burns. Their friendship and support have continued to inspire, and drive me to be the best that I can.

To my family, thank you! To Warren, you are my best friend and hubby, and although opposite in so many ways, we continue to have a shared vision and journey, and you are still my biggest fan! To Freyja and Ellowyn, you are growing into amazing young people, and I love you both so much!

Finally, I would like to thank myself! I continue to surprise myself with my resilience and love of life, despite the knock downs and challenges life brings! As a teenager in Essex, I was told I would never make it to university. I proved them wrong!

CHAPTER 1

Introduction

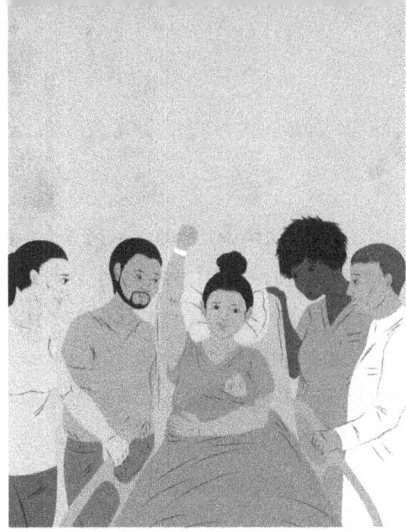

When I published my first book in 2021 my aim was to increase women's knowledge about their birthing options following a previous caesarean. I used a combination of other's and my own research undertaken for my PhD to discuss the options available. I also used storytelling, both my experiences and stories from women who had experienced a VBAC, to connect with women. My hope was that my book could help at least one woman to make an informed decision on her birth after caesarean options.

A few months after my book was published, I was contacted by a woman on social media. Let's call her Amy. At 36 weeks, Amy had a repeat caesarean booked and had been cared for by a combination of doctors and midwives in her local hospital antenatal clinic. At that later stage of her pregnancy, Amy came across my book online and read it in one go. The book was the first time she had been introduced to the option of having a VBAC and Amy realised that was the birthing option she wanted. At her next antenatal appointment, Amy arrived with the book in her bag and stated she wanted a VBAC. She received full support and had a VBAC a few weeks later. Amy told me she was so grateful for being able to read my book and the impact it had on her achieving a VBAC.

I was overjoyed in hearing her story, but I was also conflicted. How did Amy get to 36 weeks gestation without any clinician fully informing her of her options? How did they consent her for a repeat caesarean and feel confident that she was making an informed decision if she didn't know about the option of a VBAC? I wondered how to increase clinician's knowledge and confidence about better birth after caesarean, a seed for this book was planted.

The seed continued to grow as I started facilitating workshops for maternity clinicians and birth workers across Australia on supporting women planning a better birth after caesarean. These started out as book launch events but grew into entire day workshops. Using my PhD findings and my book, I facilitated interprofessional workshops attended by doulas, midwives, physiotherapists, doctors and students of these professions. I travelled across Australia and held workshops in Sydney, Wollongong, Blue Mountains, Brisbane, Gold Coast, Townsville, Perth, Adelaide, and Melbourne, and one in London, UK and Washington State, USA. I loved facilitating them. I feel I learnt as much from the participants as they did from me and the days were full of facts, research, storytelling, art, reflection, and laughter. This book is based on the workshops and the stories are from myself and participants that attended the workshops.

A little bit about me. I am a Registered Nurse and a Registered Midwife by profession. My nursing career started in the UK and led me to working in emergency, adult, paediatric, and neonatal intensive care, remote and expedition nursing, hyperbaric nursing, and disability care. As a midwife I have worked in tertiary referral hospitals, regional and small hospitals, a standalone birthing unit, and had my own private midwifery practice offering homebirths. I left the UK in 2002 with just a backpack and worked and travelled as a nurse through Malaysia and Indonesia, finally landing in Australia. I was meant to be here for 1 year and I am still here, now a citizen, 23 years later!

I have birthed two children, the first by caesarean and the second a VBAC with 13 months between births. I have written my birth stories in my previous book, *Birth after Caesarean: Your Journey to a Better Birth* so I won't repeat them here, but in summary they were both planned homebirths and both took place in hospital.

During my second pregnancy, I felt a gap in my knowledge as a midwife around planning a VBAC and I dived into reading research. Following my VBAC, I shared my story at a community forum and was approached by Professor Hannah Dahlen. Hannah encouraged me to consider doing research on VBAC and within a couple of years, whilst caring for 2 young children and 3 bonus children, I started my first higher degree in research (HDR): a Master of Nursing (Honours) into women's experiences of planning a VBAC at home. During this HDR, I fell in love with the research process and whilst my Master's thesis was being examined, I applied to commence my PhD.

I started my PhD in 2016 initially full time but was successful at the end of the first year to secure a full-time position as a Lecturer in Nursing and Midwifery at Western Sydney University, so changed to doing my PhD part time. I was warned that doing this would make it almost impossible to finish my PhD, but I set an intention to submit within the year that I would complete if I remained full time. Intentions are powerful and I submitted my PhD for examination in October 2020.

I am still at WSU as a Senior Lecturer of Midwifery, and I love my work. I get to work on midwifery research, design innovative curriculum, supervise amazing future researchers doing their own HDR's and teach the next generation of midwives and leaders. Sometimes all in one day! Over the years I have realised that writing is a creative form that I also enjoy. As an academic, this is usually in the form of peer-reviewed journal articles. I also love the free form of writing books like this one. The process allows for my mind to take mini dives into lots of interesting caves and synthesize it for you, the reader. I hope you enjoy the journeys that I go on as much as I enjoy them!

Language in Maternity Care

It is indisputable that language matters. What we say as clinicians has a positive or negative impact on women and their families. Let's look at a fictional example of the impact of language.

Most of my research has been exploring maternity care from the woman's perspective, and it has given me a unique perspective of understanding the impact of language in maternity care. Let's have a look at the following case study.

CASE STUDY 🔍

Diwata is a 28-year-old woman pregnant for the first time. She migrated to Australia from the Philippines 2 years ago and lives with her husband. All her family are still in the Philippines. From a clinical viewpoint, her pregnancy has been uneventful, she has attended the standard antenatal clinic regularly, and her measurements and observations are within normal parameters. At her 36-week appointment a midwife mentions to her the possibility that the baby might not fit through her pelvis as she is short and her white husband is tall, even though her fundus measurement is correct for her gestation.

At 38 weeks, a doctor informs her about an induction of labour and told that it is routine to perform an induction at 40 weeks for women from Southeast Asia, although no explanation is given why. Two weeks later Diwata is being induced. Diwata wanted to be upright and active in labour but is told by the midwife on duty that she won't be able to cope with the pain of an induced labour and encouraged to get an early epidural. This causes Diwata to be restricted to her bed for many hours, and following one of the epidural top ups, the foetal heart rate starts having decelerations that are becoming slower to reach the baseline. Diwata has a vaginal examination and is told she is still "6 centimetres" dilated, and the head is still high. The doctor "consents" Diwata for a caesarean stating that she was a failed induction, and her pelvis was too small for the baby's head to descend.

REFLECTION

What did you get from this example case study?

- Does this sound like a routine case study to you?
- Does the outcome of a caesarean sound likely to you?
- Can you identify any biases in her care?

How do you think Diwata would reflect on this experience?

- What would she take away from this birthing experience?
- How will this impact her next birth after caesarean?

Diwata has some challenges–she is a migrant to Australia and has no family here. She may be able to have contact with them, but she is certainly vulnerable to family and cultural isolation. At 36 weeks, she experiences racial bias regarding her mixed-race marriage. Cephalopelvic disproportion (CPD) may be a concern for the midwife, but how does that come across to the Diwata? Maybe she has received negative reactions from her or her husband's family or community about her marriage and this language affirms these beliefs. The racial profiling continues when Diwata is told she needs to be induced at 40 weeks due to the region she was born in. Then look at the language she takes away as the reasons for caesarean–she failed labour and her pelvis was too small. Maybe she also felt a loss of control from the whole experience. Diwata would enter motherhood with feelings of failure in her body and a lack of autonomy. How do you think this will impact her mothering journey?

Unfortunately, women are adept at absorbing criticism about their bodies, and many have received body shaming comments from a young age. Body shaming can be intentionally negative or intentionally innocuous. In the case study of Diwata, the clinician's intention for stating her pelvis was too small may have been to add a level of explanation. However, the impact was to shame Diwata's body.

> *Body shaming is a form of social aggression. It is a body-specific subtype of appearance teasing, often occurring online. Body shaming is an umbrella term for other, more specific concepts such as fat-shaming, thin/skinny-shaming, etc. When intentional, malevolent forms of (online) body shaming are repeatedly expressed by the same perpetrator(s), body shaming turns into a form of cyberbullying. In the context of trolling, (online) body shaming can also be a tactic/tool for trolls to provoke answers of the victim* (Schlüter et al., 2023, p. 33).

As clinicians we often use terms seen in research studies without a thought to the impact of the language. Relevant to birth after caesarean are the following terms:

- Trial of labour / scar
- Successful / Failed VBAC

As a researcher into women's experiences of maternity care, I believe these terms are problematic. The term "trial of labour or scar" denotes the woman (or only her scar) being given an opportunity to "try-out" labour with the knowledge that she may prove unworthy and fail the try-out. A different imagery, described in the book *The Silent Knife*, is that the woman is put on trial. It is the judge who slams down their gavel and convicts her as guilty of failing her attempt of a VBAC, and commits her to a repeat caesarean (Cohen & Estner, 1983). It also assumes that having a repeat caesarean after planning a VBAC is inherently negative. These imageries denote the woman as the subservient person with no control over their options and the clinicians as the decision makers. There is a significant power imbalance in the language.

The other terms I find problematic are "successful vs failed VBAC." As we will discuss in the next chapter, internationally VBAC rates are low, and most women have repeat caesareans. Therefore, for every woman who has a "successful" VBAC, there are many more who have a "failed" VBAC. How would being classified as a "failed VBAC" impact a woman? I can imagine this wouldn't be the first time she would have heard the "failed" narrative.

The language I use in this book is simple, factual, and not emotive, and I encourage you to use them in your clinical and research practice.

- Planning /planned a VBAC
- Planning /planned a repeat caesarean
- Had a VBAC
- Had a repeat caesarean (before or during labour)

I would also like to acknowledge that I use the term "woman" through-out this book. I recognise that individuals have diverse gender identities. I choose to use the term "woman/women" in recognition that interna-tionally women remain oppressed and marginalised, and in maternity care can be subjected to gendered violence due to patriarchal systems and practices. By using the term "woman/women" I do not wish to exclude individuals who give birth and don't identify as women. You are welcome here if you identify as non-binary, male, woman, and any other identity that describes you. Be proud to be you!

Introducing the Content of This Book

The aim of this book is to increase your confidence in supporting women to have better births after a previous caesarean. I will use current research to explore the issues surrounding birth after caesarean. I will also use my own research from my PhD, and other studies, to inform the use of the four factors framework for supporting better births after caesarean. I include the experiences of other clinicians to explore how they support women to have better births after caesarean.

Throughout the book you will also find quotes from women in speech boxes with the instagram sign in them.. When I was writing this book, I reached out on social media for advice they would give health care professionals on how best to support their planning their better birth after caesarean. They are also included in the final chapter. We must always centre the voice and experience of women when we are providing respectful maternity care.

Finally, there will also be reflection points throughout the book to remind you to stop and reflect on the information you have read and some questions to help guide your reflective practice.

CHAPTER 2

History, Policies, and Rates

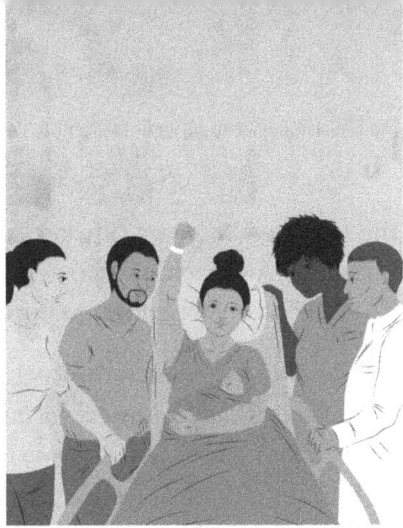

One thing must always be borne in mind, viz., that no matter how carefully a uterine incision is sutured, we can never be certain that the cicatrized uterine wall will stand a subsequent pregnancy and labor without rupture. This means the usual rule is, *once a Caesarean always a Caesarean*. Edwin B. Cragin, M.D. (Cragin, 1916)

Historical Changes to Caesarean Section

One hundred and eight years ago, Dr Edwin Cragin wrote the words in the *New York Medical Journal* that became known as the Dictum of Cragin, "once a caesarean, always a caesarean" (Todman, 2007). This view became entrenched in medical and societal views around birth after caesarean. Surprisingly, the view is still held by many clinicians in the maternity space today. In this chapter I will explore the changes that have occurred to allow this belief to be disregarded and replaced with the statement "VBAC is a safe birthing option for the majority of women."

Caesarean sections are one of the oldest recorded surgeries. In ancient times the operation was a last resort performed on dying or dead women in attempt to save the baby. The operation was sanctioned by the Christian church in the Middle Ages to separate the baby from the mother to allow for a baptism and burial (Rucker & Rucker, 1951; Todman, 2007).

The first book on caesareans was published by the Duke of Savoy's physician, Francois Rousset, in 1588, and reported on 15 cases over the previous 80 years (Rucker & Rucker, 1951). It included the case of Elisabeth Alespachin, who was operated on by her husband, Jacob Nufer, a Swiss sow gelder. As described by J.P. Boley (1935):

> *For days she had severe labour pains. The combined skill of a dozen midwives and barbers did not avail to deliver the patient. As there was no longer any hope of relieving her, the husband said that if she would have confidence in him, he would undertake an operation, which, by the grace of God, might possibly succeed. His wife replied that she would undergo anything to be relieved. The authorities at first turned a deaf ear to the husband's petition for permission to carry this out, but he was not one to take "No" for an answer. Returning with authority, he told the patient's attendants that those having sufficient courage might remain in the room with him, otherwise they must clear out. After imploring Divine aid, he laid his wife on a table, incised the abdominal wall, then the uterus, after which he quickly extracted the child. Several sutures were placed in the abdominal wall. The wound healed and the woman lived to be 77, and was able to bear several children, even twins, in the usual way, one of the children becoming a judge* (Boley, 1935, p. 557).

Caesareans at this time didn't include suturing to the uterus as they would have required removal. Instead, the belief was the uterus wound would heal through the contraction process. This contributed to the high rates of maternal morbidity due to haemorrhage and infection (Boley, 1935; Todman, 2007). It wasn't until 1880s that German obstetricians documented their methods of using sutures made of silver wire to close the uterine wound. The material was developed and used by J. Marion Sims to treat fistulas from traumatic childbirth (Sims, 1886). The greater understanding and development of anaesthetics, aseptic techniques, and suturing resulted in reduced maternal mortality and increased use of caesareans on living women.

Although there had been some development in surgical techniques from a vertical to a lower transverse incision of the abdomen, and later fascia, and to repairing in layers, there wasn't use of a transverse incision on the uterus until 1926. James Munro Kerr, a Professor of Obstetrics from Glasgow developed the Kerr transverse incision technique, yet it didn't gain widespread acceptance till the 1940s (Todman, 2007). The transverse incision on the uterus resulted in less haemorrhage and decreased uterine ruptures in subsequent pregnancies (Lurie & Glezerman, 2003). There have been many more advances in surgical, anaesthetic and aseptic techniques in the decades since and this has resulted in caesarean sections becoming a relatively safe and increasingly common operation in high-resource settings.

At this point, I would like to acknowledge the silent voices of the women throughout history for whom these various techniques were tested on. Their names and their experiences of maternity care are not recorded, and the techniques are named after the men who perfected them, not the women who were subjected to them, many of whom were enslaved Black women. As a woman who has benefited from the progress in caesarean section techniques, I honour and remember the many women who went before me.

To revisit the Dictum of Cragin, it appears that he mentions sutures on the uterus. However, there is no reference to the type of uterine incision. It is likely he was still using a longitudinal incision on the uterus. I suggest we recognise the dictum within the context it was written, and as a collective consciously remember the phrase is over 100 years out of date!

Impact of VBAC Policies

In this section, I delve into the historical evolution of policies surrounding VBAC in the United States of America (USA) and its consequential impact on guidance and support for VBAC in Australia and globally. The trajectory begins with Cohen and Estner's seminal work in 1983, which traced the increasing support for VBAC from the 1940s to the 1980s in the USA (Cohen & Estner, 1983). Despite positive outcomes reported during this period, the caesarean rates continued to rise.

The 1980s marked a pivotal time, with the National Institute of Health (NIH) endorsing VBAC due to safety concerns and the escalating caesarean rates (Placek & Taffel, 1988). However, by 1984, the caesarean rate had surged to 21.1%. The American College of Obstetricians and Gynecologists (ACOG) released guidelines in 1985, advocating for VBAC, but imposing stringent provisions including *"24-hour blood banking, continuous EFM (electronic fetal monitoring), patient blood screening, immediate presence (throughout the entire labor) of a physician capable of performing a C-section, on-site anaesthesia coverage, and the ability to move from decision to incision within 30 minutes"* (Placek & Taffel, 1988, p. 514).

In 1995, ACOG recommended VBAC for women with a previous caesarean, given the absence of medical complications (Gregory et al., 2010). Despite initial optimism, a backlash ensued after two systematic reviews raised adverse findings and medico-legal concerns, prompting a revised ACOG guideline in 1999 (Roberts, 2007; Zweifler et al., 2006). This guideline emphasised the need for immediate availability of resources for emergency caesarean, resulting in a significant reduction in facilities offering VBAC across the USA, especially small and rural hospitals (Barger et al., 2013). By 2004, the VBAC rate had plummeted to 9.2% (Roberts, 2007).

The impact extended beyond the USA, influencing professional organisations globally, despite the guidelines lacking high-level evidence (Foureur, 2010). Concurrently, the growing medical-legal concerns led to a decline in VBAC availability (Cunningham et al., 2010), with a survey indicating that 26% of obstetricians in the USA ceased offering VBAC due to fear of litigation (Klagholz & Strunk, 2009).

In 2010, the NIH published a report advocating a review of the recommendation for immediate availability due to the diminishing VBAC rates and insufficient evidence supporting its benefit (Cunningham et al., 2010). However, subsequent ACOG guidelines in 2010 maintained the emphasis on immediate availability (ACOG, 2010).

International guidelines remained relatively unchanged from 2010 until 2017. Notable shifts occurred with the release of updated ACOG and National Institute of Health and Care Excellence (NICE) guidelines in 2017 and 2019, respectively. The ACOG guidelines granted most women with a previous low-transverse incision the right to plan for a VBAC, considering various factors (ACOG, 2017). Meanwhile, NICE recommended against routinely offering intravenous cannulas during labour, and expanded analgesic options (NICE., 2019). The UK guidelines acknowledged the lack of evidence comparing continuous foetal monitoring to intermittent auscultation for women planning a VBAC (Dunning et al., 2019). The Royal Australian and New Zealand College of Obstetricians and Gynaecologists (RANZCOG) guidelines were also updated in March 2019, with no changes in the document from the 2015 version and without reference to the updated ACOG guideline of 2017 (RANZCOG, 2019b).

In summary, the historical landscape of VBAC policies, particularly in the USA, has undergone dynamic changes, impacting health care providers globally and shaping the options available to women seeking VBAC.

REFLECTION

Was there anything from the history of caesareans that you found interesting?

- How will you respond to an individual that states "once a caesarean, always a caesarean" now?

What do the latest professional college/health department guidelines in your country say about birth after a previous caesarean?

- Are they based on current evidence?
- Do they consider the woman's perspective/experience?

VBAC Rates

The cumulative impact of the various policy changes has resulted in low VBAC rates in many countries, however there are variations internationally.

In this section I explore international caesarean and VBAC rates. Firstly, I want to give an explanation on the VBAC rates that are reported. There is a fundamental difference between VBAC rates based on population data and VBAC rates reported in studies and the difference is having data on the *intention* of mode of birth.

For example, in the *Australian Mothers and Babies* report, they give a VBAC rate in 2022 as 13% for women with one previous caesarean (AIHW, 2024). That means 13% of all the women who had one previous caesarean and birthed in 2022 had a VBAC. There were 3.7% of women who had a forceps or instrumental birth and 83.2% of women had a repeat caesarean. From that data, we know neither the *intention* of the woman nor what mode of birth her plan was. For example, how many of the 83.2% of women having a caesarean planned a VBAC and had a repeat caesarean or how many planned a caesarean outright?

In research studies, the VBAC rate is based on knowing the *intention* of mode of birth. Let's look at a small study where I was part of the research team. This study looked at the outcomes for women planning a VBAC at a private hospital in Australia. In this retrospective cohort study:

> There were 322 (15.8%) women from a total of 2039 individuals who planned a VBAC, and of these, 148 (46.0%) had a completed VBAC. Of the women who had a VBAC, 80 (54.1%) had a normal vaginal birth, and 68 (45.9%) had an instrumental vaginal birth (Chu et al., 2024, p. 3&4).

There were 84.2% of women who planned and had a repeat caesarean. This resulted in a completed VBAC rate of 46% (inclusive of instrumental birth). Some studies use different terminology such as successful VBAC/TOLAC but I have already discussed why this language is problematic (see chapter 1).

International Caesarean Section and VBAC Rates

In the USA, the caesarean rate has remained consistent at 31-32% from 2013 to 2023. However, there are variations in rates depending on the State. In 2023, there was a caesarean rate of 24% in Alaska compared to a rate of 39% in Mississippi (National Center for Health Statistics, 2025a). The VBAC rate in the USA was reported as 13.3% in 2018 (Osterman, 2020) and has increased to 15% in 2023 (National Center for Health Statistics, 2025b).

In the UK caesarean rates continued to increase from 25% in 2013/14 to 38% in 2022/23 (Office for Health Improvement and Disparities, 2025). In the 2015 European Perinatal statistics, the UK had a VBAC rate that ranged from 16% in Scotland, 21.6% in Northern Ireland, 22.6% in Wales and 27% in England (Euro-Peristat Project, 2018).

Across Europe there is variation in caesarean rates with an average of 27% from a reported range of 2015-2019, ranging from Norway with 16% to Cyprus with 57% (Euro-Peristat Project, 2022).

There is also great variation in VBAC rates in Europe with a median of 26%, with Finland having the highest rate of 55.4% and Cyprus with a rate of 4.7% (Euro-Peristat Project, 2018).

In Australia, the caesarean rate has increased from 32% in 2010 to 39% in 2022 and the VBAC rate for women who had one previous caesarean was 13% in 2022 (AIHW, 2024).

A meta-analysis of pooled data from across Eastern Africa found a caesarean rate of 24%, ranging from 12% in Uganda to 28% in Ethiopia (Habteyes et al., 2024). There is a lack of reportable population data on VBAC rates.

It is beyond the scope of this book to map the caesarean and VBAC rates of 195 countries, and for many countries this data is neither recorded nor available. It is important to note that there is a global increase in caesareans that is projected to increase to 29% by 2030 (Angolile et al., 2023). The USA, UK, much of Europe, and Australia have surpassed this projected rate already. The rise in caesarean rates inevitably leads to a rise in women planning their next birth after caesarean. All these women need and deserve committed clinicians who will support them to have their best birth after caesareans.

CHAPTER 3

The Risk/Benefits of Birth after Caesarean Options

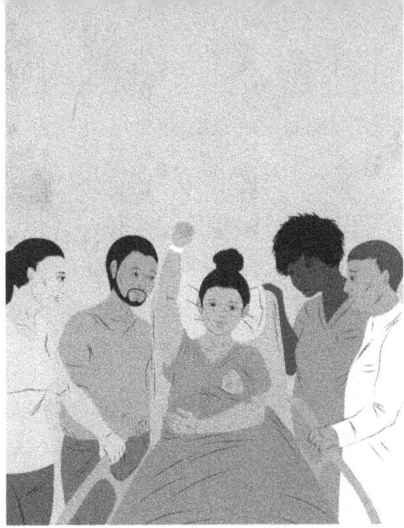

This chapter looks at the statistics around birth after caesarean options using current research. The chapter also explores uterine rupture using current research: what increases uterine rupture rates, interpregnancy intervals, and multiple caesareans. This chapter also explores the issues associated with having repeat and multiple caesareans, such as placental adhesion abnormalities, and caesarean and perineal wound complications.

Uterine Rupture

Uterine rupture is the most identified risk of planning a VBAC. As a clinician, you are aware of that risk, and may have cared for a woman who has had a uterine rupture in the past. It is important to revisit the data around uterine rupture to ensure that the information given to women and their families is based on current evidence, rather than fear.

A uterine rupture can be described as a separation through all three layers of the uterus. These layers are the endometrium (inner epithelial layer), myometrium (smooth muscle layer) and perimetrium (serosal outer surface) (Togioka & Tonismae, 2021), and exposing through to the abdominal cavity (Xie et al., 2024). Uterine rupture can occur during pregnancy or labour in women without a scar on their uterus, and more commonly, in women with a scar due to previous uterine surgery, such as caesarean and myomectomy.

An international study of 270 women who had uterine ruptures during pregnancy found 82.9% of women had a previous uterine surgical history. The ruptures occurred more frequently after 37 weeks gestation (Tinelli et al., 2022).

A uterine dehiscence or partial rupture is an incomplete separation that does not involve all three layers of the uterus.

> *Uterine dehiscence can produce a uterine window – a thinning of the uterine wall that may allow the foetus to be seen through the myometrium* (Togioka & Tonismae, 2021, p. 1).

A dehiscence can be naturally occurring and incidental and can be found during a repeat caesarean during labour.

Uterine rupture is a very rare occurrence and rupture rates are less than 1%, let's have a look at some of the large population studies. The International Network of Obstetric Survey Systems Study (INOSS) of uterine rupture is one of the most comprehensive studies on this complication. This multinational, population-based research examined data from 2,625,017 births across nine European countries between 2004 and 2014 (Vandenberghe et al., 2019). Among these births, 864 cases of complete uterine rupture were identified, resulting in a prevalence of 3.3 per 10,000 births (0.03%). There were 331,925 women who had a history of a previous caesarean and 743 of these women that had a uterine rupture, resulting in an increased rupture rate of 22 per 10,000 births (0.22%).

A study from China included 209,112 births between 2013 and 2020 identified 41 cases of complete and partial uterine rupture resulting in a prevalence of 1.96 per 10,000 (0.019%) (Wan et al., 2022). There were 37% of complete uterine ruptures out of the 41 cases. From the 41 cases there were 28 women who had a history of previous caesarean; however, the authors didn't publish the number of women who had a previous caesarean from the included 209,112 births.

Let's now focus on the maternal and neonatal outcomes of the uterine rupture from these studies. The INOSS study by Vandenberghe et al. (2019) reported 864 cases of uterine rupture. Among these women,

21% required blood transfusions exceeding four units of packed red blood cells, 20% necessitated intensive care unit admission, and 10% underwent hysterectomy. Tragically, two maternal deaths occurred, highlighting a 0.2% maternal mortality rate.

Neonatal outcomes found 28% of infants experiencing asphyxia and a 10% neonatal mortality rate. However, it's crucial to contextualise these findings. The overall perinatal morbidity rate of 0.03% in this cohort is comparable to the Australian neonatal death rate for pregnancies beyond 36 weeks gestation, which stands at 0.05% (AIHW, 2024).

In the Wan et al. (2022) study in China, 39% of the 41 women with a uterine rupture had maternal and/or neonatal complications. There were 31% of women who had a postpartum haemorrhage. The neonatal outcomes included 12% of NICU admissions and 3 cases of neonatal death (7%).

To summarise let's look at the INNOS study as we know the number of women in their cohort who had a previous caesarean.

- **Women with a previous caesarean:** 334,652
- **Uterine ruptures:** 743
- **Uterine rupture rate:** 0.22%
- **Maternal fatalities:** 2 (0.2% of women who had a rupture)
- **Perinatal mortalities:** 0.03% (10% of babies from uterine rupture)

In conclusion, while the risk of uterine rupture during attempted vaginal birth after caesarean (VBAC) remains present, it is generally low. Maternal mortality following uterine rupture is rare, particularly with prompt access to emergency medical care. Furthermore, a high proportion (90%) of infants survive uterine rupture.

Identifying a Uterine Rupture

A few studies have retrospectively looked at the onset and features of a uterine rupture. Guiliano et al. (2014) looked at 52 partial and complete uterine ruptures and found several signs and symptoms were experienced and these have also been found in the studies by Markou et al. (2017) and Chang (2020). Wan et al. (2022) also looked at the 41 cases of uterine rupture and Dimitrova et al. (2022) explored 92 cases of complete uterine rupture. Tinelli et al. (2021) looked at the presentation of uterine rupture during pregnancy in 270 women. These are listed in table 1.

TABLE 1: SIGNS OF UTERINE RUPTURE

Sign / Symptom	Guiliano et al. (2014) n=52	Chang et al. (2020) n=18	Markou et al. (2017) n=126	Wan et al. (2022) n=41	Dimitrova et al. (2022) N=29	Tinelli et al. (2021) n=270
Fetal heart rate abnormality	46%	78%	47%	42%	62%	6%
Abdominal pain	25%	28%	48%	56%	31%	31%
Vaginal bleeding	23%	33%	30%	32%	-	13%
Loss of presentation	15%	-	-	-	-	-
Haematuria	4%	11%	-	-	-	-
Asymptomatic	33%	11%	-	-	10%	-
Atony	-	-	-	-	36%	-
Other	-	-	-	12%	-	12%

* - These were not reported on in the study

The most common clinical manifestations of uterine rupture during labour include foetal heart rate (FHR) abnormalities, particularly persistent bradycardia (Guiliano et al., 2014), abdominal pain beyond typical labour contractions, and abnormal vaginal bleeding. The recognition of FHR abnormalities as a critical sign of uterine rupture underscores the inclusion of continuous cardiotocography (CTG) monitoring during VBAC, as outlined in current guidelines from ACOG and RANZCOG (ACOG, 2019; RANZCOG, 2019a).

While intermittent auscultation using a Doppler may detect some FHR abnormalities, its effectiveness in identifying the subtle changes associated with uterine rupture remains uncertain. A large Cochrane review comparing continuous CTG monitoring to intermittent auscultation found no significant difference in neonatal mortality but revealed higher rates of interventions, including caesareans, with continuous monitoring (Alfirevic et al., 2017).

Following a Uterine Rupture

If a woman has experienced a uterine rupture but proceeds to have another pregnancy, she must consider the potential outcomes of their next pregnancy. Few studies have investigated the obstetric outcomes in women with a history of uterine rupture or dehiscence. One US study examined 60 women (20 with prior rupture, 40 with prior dehiscence), all of whom underwent repeat elective caesarean, primarily between 36- and 39-weeks gestation. A dehiscence rate of 6.7% was observed in this cohort (Fox et al., 2014).

Long-term follow-up of these women revealed a 12% rate of dehiscence and a 1% rate of recurrent uterine rupture in subsequent pregnancies (Fox, 2020).

A more recent study from Denmark, published in 2022, explored the outcomes of 70 women with a previous complete uterine rupture in their subsequent birth and compared their outcomes to 126 women with no previous uterine rupture (Thisted et al., 2022). All women's previous births had been via caesarean. The women with a previous uterine rupture had a uterine rupture rate in their subsequent birth of 8.6% compared to 0.8% of women without a previous uterine rupture and there were statistically significantly more babies that required CPAP in the previous uterine rupture group.

Both Fox (2020) and Thisted et al. (2022) recommended that women with a previous uterine rupture or dehiscence should have a repeat elective caesarean before the onset of spontaneous labour, or early in labour, at no later than 37 to 38 weeks gestation. There are no published studies that compare the outcomes of women with a previous complete or partial uterine rupture who have a vaginal birth compared to having a caesarean.

A vital aspect that is missing from this research is the voice and experience of women. There is very little research on women's experiences of planning a VBAC after a rupture (VBAR) but there are women who wish to have this experience. In my previous book, Kari Lammer from Iowa, USA, shared her experience of a VBAR. I currently supervise a Master of Research student exploring women's experiences of having a previous uterine rupture and their subsequent pregnancy. I look forward to seeing what Ashlee finds from interviewing women with this experience. This research is going to be vital to ensure women's voices are heard and their wishes and choices are centred.

Birth after Caesarean Modes of Birth

Research examining birth outcomes after caesarean delivery has histori-cally presented data based on the intended mode of birth: planned-vaginal birth after caesarean (VBAC) versus planned repeat caesarean section. This approach, while seemingly straightforward, can be misleading. A significant proportion of women initially planning VBAC ultimately undergo a repeat caesarean. This discrepancy between intended and actual birth modes can skew the results and create an inaccurate picture of the true risks and benefits associated with each mode of birth.

Early studies, such as Crowther (2012) and those by Gilbert (2012) and Macones et al. (2005), primarily relied on this "intended mode" analysis. For example, Crowther (2012) observed lower rates of adverse fetal and infant outcomes in the planned-repeat-caesarean group compared to the planned-VBAC group. However, this comparison is incomplete. Only 43% of women in the planned-VBAC group achieved vaginal birth. The remaining women experienced either elective or emergency caesareans, effectively diluting the outcomes within the planned-VBAC group and potentially skewing the results in favour of planned repeat caesarean.

Studies that analyse outcomes based on the actual mode of birth provide a more accurate and clinically relevant picture and allows for a more meaningful comparison for women of outcomes across different birth pathways. Women are able to understand that planning a VBAC may result in a repeat caesarean and want to know what the outcomes could be for all three of modes of birth: VBAC, planned VBAC resulting in a repeat caesarean, and a repeat planned caesarean.

However, even using this method of reporting, challenges remain. Inconsistency in the reported outcomes across different studies, includ-ing variations in the specific outcomes measured, the definitions used, and the inclusion criteria, complicates the synthesis of evidence and hinders clear comparisons.

Table 2 summarises the key findings from these studies, highlighting statis-tically significant differences. It is crucial to remember that statistically significant differences indicate that the observed results are unlikely to be due to chance. However, clinical significance, or the practical importance of these differences for care, must also be carefully considered.

TABLE 2: OUTCOMES BETWEEN MODE OF BIRTH

Study	Planned CS	Planned VBAC had CS	VBAC
Pont et al. (2018)	Requiring a blood transfusion		
	0.3%	1.2%	1.4%
Takeya et al. (2020)	Postpartum Haemorrhage (PPH)		
	26%	20%	8%
Fitzpatrick et al. (2019)	Uterine rupture		
	0.04%	0.74%	0.04%
	Blood transfusion		
	0.5%	1.37%	1.05%
	Sepsis (Major infection)		
	0.17%	0.48%	0.18%	
	Other infections		
	2.23%	4.29%	1.53%
	Exclusive breastfeeding at 6 to 8 weeks		
	24.94%	33.53%	33.57%
	Adverse outcome for baby		
	6.37%	10.33%	7.06%

In conclusion, while some research has evolved towards more robust methodologies, the complexities of comparing birth outcomes after caesarean remain. Clinicians must carefully interpret the available evidence, considering the limitations of different study designs and the potential impact of confounding factors. A comprehensive understanding of the risks and benefits associated with each mode of birth is essential for providing women with informed and individualised support.

Table 2 identifies differences across modes of birth. These findings are supported by large-scale population studies: Pont et al. (2018) analysed data from 90,439 women in New South Wales, Australia; Takeya et al. (2020) examined 34,460 women in Japan; and Fitzpatrick et al. (2019) reviewed data from 74,043 women in Scotland. Importantly, the absolute rates of these outcomes across all groups remain relatively low.

While the rates of most adverse outcomes are generally highest in the planned caesarean cohort, there are higher postpartum haemorrhage rates in the planned caesarean cohort reported by Takeya et al. (2020) and lower rates of exclusive breastfeeding at 6-8 weeks in the planned caesarean cohort observed by Fitzpatrick et al. (2019).

It's crucial to acknowledge that these statistical analyses provide only a partial picture. Most importantly, these studies do not capture the experiences of women following each birth mode. Understanding the psychological and emotional impact of different birth experiences is vitally important and will be explored further in subsequent chapters.

Complications Following Caesarean and VBAC

Abnormalities of Placentation

Uterine anatomy consists of three layers: the perimetrium (outer layer), the myometrium (thick muscular layer), and the endometrium (inner mucosal layer) (Pairman et al., 2022).

Placenta accreta spectrum (PAS) refers to a range of conditions where the placenta abnormally attaches to the uterine wall. As described in an expert review of PAS:

PAS is a congenital placental disorder secondary to the permanent remodeling of the uterine wall, which essentially occurs after surgery of the lower segment (Jauniaux et al., 2022, p. 389). The review explains that:

It is the size of the scar defect, the amount of placental tissue developing inside the scar, and the residual myometrial thickness in the scar area that determine the distance between the placental basal plate and the uterine serosa and thus the risk of accreta placentation (Jauniaux et al., 2022, p. 384).

The incidence of PAS has risen particularly in conjunction with increasing caesarean rates (Matsuzaki et al., 2021). Due to the abnormal placental implantation, women with PAS are at higher risk of surgical morbidity and mortality such as postpartum haemorrhage , often requiring blood transfusions and potentially necessitating a hysterectomy (Matsuzaki et al., 2021).

The risk of PAS increases with each subsequent caesarean delivery. After one prior caesarean, the risk is approximately 3%. This risk escalates to 11% after two caesareans, 40% after three, 60% after four, and 67% after five or more caesareans (Sandall et al., 2018).

Adhesions

Abdominal/pelvic adhesions are fibrous, band-like structures that form between abdominal organs or between the peritoneum and abdominal wall when trauma induces inflammation and disrupts normal tissue (Lyell, 2011, p. S11).

Caesarean delivery can lead to the formation of adhesions within the abdomen and pelvis. These adhesions can cause chronic abdominal or pelvic pain, pain during bowel movements, and dyspareunia (painful sexual intercourse) (Wasserman et al., 2018). Peritoneal wound healing can be complicated by the inflammatory response of the body and adhesion formation results from an excessive inflammatory response. It has been suggested that women with chronic inflammatory disorders, including obesity, are at an increased risk of adhesion formation following caesareans (Kinay et al., 2022).

Pelvic adhesions can increase the risk of secondary infertility and ectopic pregnancy. Subsequent caesareans in women with adhesions may be associated with increased surgical complications and higher rates of infection (Saban et al., 2019).

A prospective study from Egypt of 300 women with a history of a previous caesarean, and who had a repeat caesarean, found 62% of women had moderate-to-severe adhesions diagnosed at the repeat caesarean (Aboshama et al., 2023). The women with moderate-to-severe adhesions experienced longer surgical time, had increased postoperative pain and complications, and delayed ambulation and bowel movements following their repeat caesarean. Women with moderate-to-severe adhesions also reported chronic pelvic pain, and raised or keloid scarring of their previous caesarean prior to their repeat caesarean.

Women experiencing chronic abdominal or pelvic pain following caesarean delivery should consult with their health care provider. Treatment options may include soft tissue mobilisation, physical therapy, medication, and manual scar therapy (Wasserman et al., 2018). Manual scar therapy can include manual scar manipulation, massage, cupping, dry needling, and taping (Lubczyńska et al., 2023).

Impact of Caesarean Delivery on Infants and Children

Emerging evidence suggests a potential link between caesarean delivery (CD) and long-term adverse health outcomes in children. Research suggests an increased risk of immune-related disorders in children born via caesarean, including obesity, type 1 diabetes mellitus, and asthma (Hoang et al., 2021). This may be attributed to disruptions in the infant gut microbiome, a phenomenon known as dysbiosis, which has been observed following caesarean (Hoang et al., 2021).

A US study involving 22,690 children observed a significantly higher incidence of otitis media and respiratory infections in those born via caesarean compared to vaginal birth. However, no significant difference in food allergy rates was noted (Kikuchi et al., 2020).

A small Czech study demonstrated that 5-year-old children born vaginally exhibited higher cognitive development scores compared to those born via caesarean, particularly in boys (Blazkova et al., 2020). However, a systematic review of seven studies found inconsistent evidence regarding the association between caesarean and lower cognitive functioning (Blake et al., 2021).

These findings highlight the need for further research to investigate the potential long-term impact of caesareans on infant and child health.

Caesarean and Perineal Wound Complications

Following caesarean, women are at risk of developing surgical site infections (SSI). An international systematic review found a pooled SSI prevalence following caesarean as 5.63% which was higher in the African region (11.91%) and lower in the Northern American region (3.87%) (Farid Mojtahedi et al., 2023). Other surgical wound complications include dehiscence, hyper granulation, peri wound maceration, scarring and medical adhesive-related skin injury (MARSI) (Rastas, 2023).

A delay in treating postoperative infections can lead to sepsis (Dong et al., 2024). Long-term complications include adhesions and scar defects, which can lead to abnormal uterine bleeding, secondary infertility, and chronic pelvic or abdominal pain (Antoine & Young, 2021; Dong et al., 2024; Hsu et al., 2022).

Women who have a VBAC risk sustaining severe perineal trauma (a third- or fourth-degree perineal tear). In Australia around 3% of women who birth vaginally experience severe perineal trauma, increasing to 4.3% for nulliparous women (AIHW, 2024). The long-term impact of experiencing a severe perineal tear can include mental health issues, relationship issues, alongside anal incontinence, perineal pain, and dsypareunia (Edqvist et al., 2022; Molyneux et al., 2024).

Studies that have compared women having a VBAC to primiparous women have found increased rates of severe perineal trauma for women who had a VBAC (Uebergang et al., 2022), however there is a lack of evidence to explain why this could occur. An Australian study found 7.1% of women who had a VBAC experienced severe perineal trauma compared to 5.7% of primiparous women (Uebergang et al., 2022).

A Swedish study found the rate of severe perineal trauma for women who had a VBAC as 12.3% compared to nulliparous women at 7% (Elvander et al., 2019). Elvander et al. (2002) found that women having a VBAC were 1.75 times more likely to experience severe tearing of the perineum compared to nulliparous women. However, when the researchers considered factors like the mother's age, height, how long the pregnancy lasted, her birth position, and the baby's size, the risk for the VBAC group was slightly lower, at 1.42 times higher. Birthing in the lithotomy position increases the risk of severe perineal trauma (Elvander et al., 2015). However, Elvander et al. (2002) found only 12.9% of women who had a VBAC birthed in an upright position compared to 20.7% of nulliparous women, which may have impacted the rate of severe perineal trauma.

Conclusion

Caesarean delivery is a major abdominal surgical procedure with potential short- and long-term physical complications for women, including the risk of placenta accreta and the development of adhesions. These complications can significantly impact women's quality of life and may have implications for subsequent pregnancies. For women who have a VBAC and experience severe perineal trauma there is also potential for short- and long-term complications. It's important to recognise that these are potential risks, and not all women will experience complications following caesarean or VBAC.

Facilitators and Barriers to VBAC

In this section, I explore the evidence around the facilitators and barriers to VBAC.

Women with Increased BMI

Women with obesity (BMI ≥ 30 kg/m2) frequently encounter weight stigma and bias from health care providers, which can present as stereotyping, bullying, and even coercion within the context of maternity care (Mulherin et al., 2013; Dejoy et al., 2016). This stigmatising environment can significantly impact the decision-making process and overall birth experience for women with obesity considering a VBAC.

While some studies have reported lower VBAC rates and increased complications, particularly during emergency caesarean delivery, in women with obesity (Wilson et al., 2020; Yao et al., 2019), it's crucial to acknowledge these findings may be confounded by several factors. Notably, women with obesity may experience being classified as higher risk which may result in less midwifery care (Mei et al., 2019). In chapter 7, I explore how midwifery models of care can result in higher VBAC rates. Furthermore, the impact of weight stigma and bias on health care access and quality of care for women with obesity cannot be ignored.

The American College of Obstetricians and Gynecologists (ACOG) guidelines (ACOG, 2019) appropriately support VBAC planning for women with obesity, emphasising the importance of individualised care. However, it is essential to recognise that women with obesity are at an increased risk of certain surgical complications, such as wound infections and venous thromboembolism, following caesarean.

Addressing and mitigating weight stigma within the health care setting is paramount to ensuring equitable and respectful care for all women, regardless of their weight. This includes fostering a supportive and non-judgmental environment, promoting respectful communication between providers and women, and actively addressing any biases that may influence clinical decision-making.

Size of Baby

Some clinicians have concern for women planning a VBAC when a baby is suspected to be large for gestational age. A study from France explored the outcomes of women with a previous caesarean and a suspected estimated fetal weight as large for gestational age (eLGA) (Chamagne et al., 2023). Estimation of fetal weight was performed using sonography between 36 and 41 weeks, and defined as a fetal weight above the 90th percentile. Out of 235 women, 28% planned a repeat caesarean and 72% planned a VBAC. From the planned VBAC group, 69% had a VBAC and 31% had a repeat caesarean. There were no significant differences between women who planned a caesarean compared to women who planned a VBAC except for a raised lactate in cord blood in the planned-VBAC cohort. There were no uterine ruptures or neonatal deaths in either cohort. The current ACOG guidelines (2019) recommend that a suspected eLGA should not prohibit women from planning a VBAC.

Interpregnancy Interval

The interpregnancy interval (IPI) is defined as the time between birth and the conception of the next pregnancy. Factors influencing IPI are diverse and include previous pregnancy and birth experiences, contraceptive use, breastfeeding duration, maternal age, unintended pregnancy, changes in relationship status, socioeconomic factors, health status, and fertility. Studies have shown a longer IPI following caesarean delivery compared to spontaneous vaginal birth, although the reasons for this remain unclear (O'Neill et al., 2013). An IPI less than 18 months is associated with preterm birth and low birth rate, and less than 6 months is associated with increased uterine rupture rates (Ahlers-Schmidt et al., 2018; Stamilio, 2007).

Informed decision-making regarding subsequent pregnancies requires women to understand the potential risks and benefits associated with different IPI lengths. However, studies demonstrate a gap in women's knowledge regarding IPI following caesarean (Ahlers-Schmidt et al., 2018). Many women lack adequate information about IPI and its impli-cations for future pregnancies. Despite this knowledge gap, women often make decisions about subsequent pregnancies within a short timeframe after their previous birth. These decisions are influenced by various factors, including prior birth experiences, personal preferences, and social and emotional factors. There is a lack of current research in this area, but I am excited to share that I am a co-supervisor for a PhD student, Alison Canty, who is focusing on IPI in Australia. I look forward to the findings of her PhD study.

Empowering women to make informed decisions about their reproductive health requires open and honest communication with their health care providers, addressing knowledge gaps through educational interventions, and fostering a supportive environment that empowers women to make informed choices about their reproductive health, including their desired IPI. There also needs to be an awareness that not all pregnancies occur when planned and women's wishes for the birth after caesarean choices should still be respected. I say this from a personal perspective as the IPI for my second pregnancy was only 4 months (much quicker than planned), and I went on to have a VBAC 13 months after my caesarean!

Multiple Caesareans

While research on vaginal birth after two or more previous caesarean deliveries (VBA2C) is limited, available evidence suggests favourable outcomes. A study from Poland reported on the outcomes of 412 women who had a history of two previous caesareans (Modzelewski et al., 2019). There were 35 (8%) of this cohort that planned a VBA2C, and 22 of these women had a VBAC. Importantly, women who had a VBA2C exhibited lower rates of maternal and perinatal morbidity compared to those who had a planned or emergency repeat caesarean (Modzelewski et al., 2019).

A study from the USA comparing 82 women planning a VBA2C to women planning a repeat caesarean found a VBAC rate of 69.5% and no difference in maternal or neonatal outcomes (Horgan et al., 2022). There was one uterine rupture in the planned VBAC group and one unplanned hysterectomy in the planned repeat caesarean group

This low planning rate for VBA2C underscores the significant challenges women face in accessing support for this option. A systematic review of 17 studies involving 5,666 women planning VBAC after multiple caesareans demonstrated a VBAC rate of 71%, a uterine rupture rate of 1.36%, and comparable neonatal and maternal outcomes compared to repeat caesarean (Tahseen & Griffiths, 2010).

The ACOG guidelines (2019) acknowledges that women with a history of two previous caesareans "be candidates for Trial of Labour After Caesarean(TOLAC)".

Cahill et al. (2010) reported encouraging outcomes in a cohort of 860 women planning VBAC after three or more caesareans, with a VBAC rate of 80%, no reported uterine ruptures, and no significant differences in maternal morbidity.

Despite these favourable outcomes, women considering VBA2C after multiple caesareans often face significant barriers, including limited support from health care providers, pervasive negativity, and doubts about their bodies' ability to successfully deliver vaginally. These challenges can significantly impact a woman's decision-making process and require compassionate and informed support from health care professionals.

Multiple Pregnancy

Existing research on VBAC in women with twin pregnancies is limited. A systematic review by Shinar et al. (2019) of 10 studies reported comparable VBAC rates in women pregnant with twins compared to those with singleton pregnancies. Notably, the review observed significantly lower infection rates in the VBAC group compared to the repeat caesarean section group. While the review reported a higher perinatal mortality rate in the VBAC group, the authors attributed this finding to the increased risk of preterm birth associated with twin pregnancies. This observation, however, has not been consistently replicated in other studies. For example, Varner et al. (2007) reported high VBAC rates and low complication rates in women with multiple gestations.

An international study explored the outcomes of 236 planned VBAC of twins (Hochler et al., 2022). There were 128 in the nonvertex presentation of the second twin group, and 108 in the both-twins-presenting-vertex group, and a VBAC rate of 76.6% and 81.5%. There was one uterine rupture reported in each group with no maternal or neonatal mortality. There were no differences in obstetric or neonatal outcomes between the cohorts. The American College of Obstetricians and Gynecologists (ACOG) guidelines (2019) support the consideration of VBAC for women with twin pregnancies.

Given the limited available data, a careful individualised assessment of risks and benefits is crucial when discussing VBAC options with women expecting twins. This assessment should consider factors such as gestational age, foetal presentation, maternal medical history, and the availability of adequate midwifery, obstetrical and neonatal support and primarily, the women's preference for mode of birth.

Breech Position

Caesarean has in recent history been the standard mode of birth for women pregnant with a breech presentation baby. However, with the re-emergence of vaginal breech birth in select centres, women who have a history of a previous caesarean and experience a subsequent breech pregnancy have renewed interest in exploring vaginal breech options.

External cephalic version (ECV) is an important intervention to consider for achieving cephalic presentation in breech pregnancies. While concerns previously existed regarding ECV safety in women with previous CS, current ACOG guidelines (2019) recognise that these women are not contra-indicated for ECV, and that success rates in rotating from breech to cephalic are comparable to those in women without previous CS.

Despite these guidelines, accessing ECV may be challenging for women with previous CS due to varying levels of provider confidence and expe-rience with this procedure in this specific population. Data on VBAC in women with subsequent breech pregnancies is limited. A small German study involving 37 women with previous CS found no significant differences in maternal or neonatal outcomes between women who planned a VBAC for breech, and those who planned a repeat caesarean. The VBAC rate in this study was also comparable to that observed in women with singleton breech pregnancies without previous CS (Paul et al., 2020).

While this study provides preliminary evidence, further research with larger sample sizes is necessary to fully understand the risks and benefits of VBAC for breech presentations in women with previous CS.

Clinicians should stay aware of current evidence and guidelines regarding ECV and VBAC in women with previous CS and breech presentations. Supportive communication is essential to ensure women have access to the full range of available options and can make informed choices about their birth plan.

Special Scars

Women with uterine scars, other than lower-segment transverse scars, have additional challenges for the next birth after caesarean. These scars, including J incisions, inverted T incisions, classical scars, low-vertical incisions, upright T incisions, lower-uterine extensions, and scars secondary to prior uterine rupture, can arise due to various factors like prematurity, foetal malpresentation, prior abdominal surgery, and resource limitations during the initial caesarean delivery.

Traditionally, women with these "special scars" are recommended to have an elective repeat caesarean at 37 to 38 weeks gestation to minimise the risk of uterine rupture during labour. However, a growing number of women with special scars desire to plan a VBAC.

While data on VBAC outcomes in women with special scars is limited, particularly for scar types beyond classical incisions, existing research suggests potential considerations. A retrospective study by Bakhshi et al. (2010) compared outcomes in 122 women with classical scars undergoing repeat caesarean delivery to a control group of 7,814 women with lower-segment transverse-caesarean scar (LSTCS). The classical-scar group had higher rates of repeat classical incisions, operative time, prolonged hospital stays, ICU admissions, and uterine dehiscence (incomplete uterine wall separation) compared to the LSTCS group (Bakhshi et al., 2010). It is important to note that all women in this study underwent repeat-caesarean delivery, and no VBAC attempts were included.

Current evidence regarding VBAC safety in women with special scars, particularly those beyond classical incisions, is scarce. While small studies by Kwee et al. (2007) and Patterson et al. (2002) included women with inverted T scars who achieved successful VBAC, the sample sizes were insufficient to draw definitive conclusions.

The American College of Obstetricians and Gynecologists (ACOG) guidelines (2019) acknowledge that women with prior low-vertical incisions may be suitable candidates for VBAC due to the lack of evidence suggesting increased risk of uterine rupture or maternal morbidity. Conversely, ACOG advises against VBAC in women with prior classical scars, T incisions, or uterine rupture.

Further research is warranted to elucidate the safety and efficacy of VBAC in women with various uterine scar types alongside research on the qualitative experiences of women with special scars.

Additional Resources

"Special Scars–Special Hope," a non-profit, volunteer led organisation supporting individuals on their special scar journeys through private social media support pages, is an invaluable resource for women with a special scar. More information can be found via their website: https://specialscars.org/.

Induction of Labour

Induction of labour involves initiating labour before it begins sponta-neously. Methods include prostaglandins (used to ripen the cervix), mechanical methods, such as cervical-ripening balloons and amniot-omy (artificial rupture of membranes), and synthetic oxytocin.

In women planning a VBAC, inducing labour requires consideration due to the potential risk of uterine rupture. Studies suggest an increased risk of uterine rupture with the use of prostaglandins, particularly in combination with oxytocin (Buhimschi et al., 2005; Dekker, 2010; Stock et al., 2013). However, recent research has shown promising results with cervical-ripening balloons followed by oxytocin. One study demon-strated higher VBAC rates, and potentially lower uterine- rupture rates, with this approach compared to oxytocin alone (Secchi et al., 2021).

ACOG acknowledges that while some studies have reported a slightly increased risk of uterine rupture with synthetic oxytocin use in the VBAC population, the overall risk is small. Therefore, oxytocin augmen-tation may be considered (ACOG, 2019).

The choice of induction method should be individualised based on clinical indications for induction, and the experience and preferences of the woman. Many women who have had a previous caesarean have experienced an induction of labour, and may have found that these experiences were negative or traumatic.

As a researcher, I lead the Birth Experience Study–International Collaboration (www.birthexperiencestudy.com). In this study, we use a co-designed maternity experiences cross-sectional survey to under-stand the perinatal journey from the women's perspective. It is currently run in over 14 countries. Findings from our first Australian BESt survey found that women overwhelmingly wished to avoid an induction of labour in subsequent pregnancies, with many women feeling they were coerced into an induction without enough information to make an informed decision (Ormsby et al., 2025).

I would have been a stronger advocate for me and my baby. I wouldn't have allowed myself to be pressured into induction and I would have waited until baby was ready on her own... (ID: 2618) (Ormsby et al., 2025, p. 3).

Place of Birth

My Masters Honours research involved a qualitative study exploring women's experiences of planning a Home Birth After Caesarean (HBAC) in Australia. This topic held personal significance as I had planned an HBAC, but ultimately transferred to hospital due to the unavailability of my homebirth team.

Through interviews with 12 women who successfully achieved HBAC, a central theme emerged: "It's [a caesarean] never happening again." Participants recounted traumatic previous caesarean experiences and described their journeys towards seeking an HBAC. Navigating the health care system often involved challenging hospital policies and encountering resistance to their birth preferences. This frequently led them to seek care from private midwives, who empowered them by shifting the dialogue from "no, you can't" to "yes, you can." These women found healing and a profound sense of empowerment through their HBAC experiences, often expressing sentiments like "I felt like Superwoman" (Keedle et al., 2015).

Research supports the potential benefits of homebirth for VBAC. Studies have demonstrated higher VBAC rates in homebirth settings compared to hospital settings (Bayrampour et al., 2021; Beckmann et al., 2014; Latendresse, 2005; Parslow & Rayment-Jones, 2024). However, a population-based US study reported a slightly higher intrapartum foetal death rate in women planning HBAC (0.29%) compared to women without a previous caesarean birthing at home (0.06%), although the three deaths were not attributed to uterine rupture (Cheyney et al., 2014).

A Canadian study found an HBAC rate of 86% compared to a hospital VBAC rate of 70%, with rare adverse outcomes observed in both settings and no significant differences between home and hospital births

(Bayrampour et al., 2021). It's crucial to remember that adverse events can occur during any birth, regardless of location. Midwives are trained to recognise and manage potential complications, and facilitate timely transfers to hospital when necessary. Open and honest communication between the woman and her midwife regarding potential transfer scenarios based on location and available resources is essential.

Summary

This has been a very busy and evidence-based chapter, and well done for getting to the end of it. Whatever our profession, we are united in our standards of practice stating we must provide evidence-based, not fear-based care. This chapter has helped you update your knowledge on the evidence around birth after caesarean.

"Reframe everything–treat them the same as first-time vaginal birther. There is no difference.

- Walk through all risks AND BENEFITS for all options and approaches.

- Don't be condescending and explain the statistics (what does less than 1% really look like).

- Walk through the cascade of interventions, the connected interventions, and why they may have ended up there last time.

- LISTEN and validate their past experience, this will help you understand the source of their questions/ fears/assumptions.

- DON'T USE language that takes away her power: you can try, we will let you, we will see, TOLAC, policy is this therefore, up to the surgeon on the day, discuss that when you're here in labour, this is routine, we will do this, etc."

REFLECTION

Reflect on the information provided in this chapter.

- Has any of this evidence surprised or challenged you?
- Have you been providing evidence-based information on risks and benefits of all modes of birth when discussing them with women?
- Do you need to update the information you provide women about the risks and benefits of birth after caesarean options?

CHAPTER 4

The VBAC Calculator

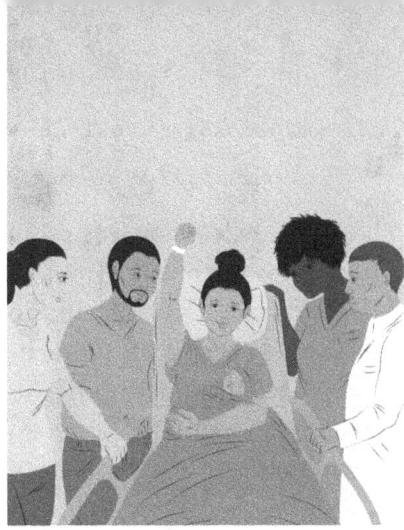

Many clinicians, especially obstetricians in the USA, use the Maternal-Fetal Medicine Units (MFMU) VBAC Success Calculator in their antenatal appointments with women who express a preference for planning a VBAC. The calculator uses a variety of data from the woman and her obstetric history to give a prediction score presented as a percentage. The prediction score tells the clinician the likelihood of a woman having a VBAC. The predictions are based on studies that have explored the facilitating factors for having a VBAC. The VBAC calculator has been validated, reproduced, adapted and tested in a variety of different languages and countries, and is available as an app for clinicians and women to use (Fagerberg et al., 2015; Lakra et al., 2020; Mooney et al., 2019).

From the outside, this calculator makes logical sense. There are greater risks to having a repeat "in-labour" caesarean compared to having a planned repeat caesarean, and not all women will have a VBAC, so let's figure out which women are more likely to have a VBAC, and those with a lower score can be actively discouraged to plan a VBAC. However, when you dig below the surface, the VBAC calculator is problematic in many ways. Let's dig into this now.

If you use the calculator, or are part of the team that designed it, please don't see this as an attack on your practice. I am writing this from my perspective as a midwife who has supported many women to have a better birth after caesarean, and as a feminist researcher that focuses on women's experiences of maternity care. I am looking at it from the women's experience through an intersectional feminist and reproductive-justice lens.

The VBAC calculator was proposed by Grobman et al. (2007). Their study reviewed the data from 7,660 women with a previous caesarean who had a subsequent birth. They found six variables that impacted VBAC rates: age, BMI, ethnicity, vaginal birth since caesarean, any history of vaginal birth and whether the reason for the caesarean was deemed as potentially recurrent (Grobman et al., 2007). Let's look at each of these.

Age

The VBAC calculator modelling found women that were younger had higher VBAC rates, and the younger the woman is, the higher they score on the calculator. Their age range is from 50 (0 points) to 15 yrs (15 points). At this point, 100 alarm bells are exploding in my head! Ageist much?

Is there any perfect age to have a baby? Young mums are subjected to so much societal and medical discrimination. In our national maternity experiences study, women under the age of 24 years experienced more birth trauma and obstetric violence (Keedle & Dahlen, 2023). You may score higher on the VBAC score, but you get treated worse in the maternity care system, and are often shunned by society (Felstead, 2020).

How about women who have worked at their career by getting tertiary education and/or working, and start having their children in their thirties? Once you hit 35 years you might get labelled as an elderly primip, or "advanced maternal age."

Is age alone enough to be included? How about the overall health of the woman? I've cared for well-resourced, health conscious, and physically fit pregnant women at a variety of ages. Many women don't have a choice about the age they are when they get pregnant, but they certainly experience the judgement if they are not within the narrow imposed 'ideal' range.

I'm not disputing the evidence around age and maternal and neonatal outcomes, but I do question the underlying bias that rewards younger age without recognition of the ongoing impact.

Boby Mass Index (BMI)

The VBAC calculator found women with a lower pre-pregnancy BMI had higher VBAC rates. The lower the BMI, the higher the score in the calculator. The VBAC calculator reaffirms weight stigma by giving less probability to women with higher BMI's and promotes decreased weight by giving higher points to women who are underweight. Women with a higher BMI (≥30 kg/m2) frequently encounter stigma and weight bias from health care professionals. A meta-ethnography of 38 studies found women with higher weight regularly felt shame, humiliation, and judgement following negative interactions with health care providers (Cunningham et al., 2024).

A study from the USA interviewing women who experienced weight stigma revealed encounters with judgment, stereotyping, bullying, and coercion within maternity care (Dejoy et al., 2016). This weight stigma, compounded by the complexities of planning a vaginal birth after caesarean, can significantly increase the pressure on women and potentially lead to disrespectful care.

While research indicates that women with higher BMIs may have lower VBAC rates, they can also experience higher complication risks in cases of emergency caesarean (Wilson et al., 2020; Yao et al., 2019). A US study of 614 women found no significant difference in VBAC rates across different weight classes, with the key factor being lower likelihood of care by a certified nurse-midwife (CNM) for women with higher BMIs (Mei et al., 2019). The ACOG guidelines emphasise that women with a BMI of 30 or more can plan a VBAC, and that their care should be individualised (ACOG, 2017).

A meta-analysis of 86 studies involving over 20 million women revealed a strong correlation between increasing maternal pre-pregnancy BMI (underweight to overweight and obesity), and a significant rise in the risk of various adverse maternal, foetal, and neonatal outcomes (Vats et al., 2021). These outcomes included an increased likelihood of caesarean, gestational diabetes, postpartum haemorrhage, pre-eclampsia, preterm premature rupture of membranes, and an elevated risk of low Apgar scores at 5 minutes, large for gestational age, and macrosomia. It also found women who were underweight had higher risk of small for gestational age and preterm birth (BMI <18.5 kg/m2).

Given the increased prevalence of surgical complications, like wound infections and venous thromboembolism, in women with higher BMIs, women with a higher weight who plan a VBAC should be supported. Clinicians need to be aware of their own weight bias, and ensure this is not influencing supporting women and providing respectful maternity care.

Ethnicity

The original VBAC calculator, originating in the USA, included African American, Hispanic, White, and Other in their predictive tool. If the woman was African American or Hispanic, they received less probability for having a VBAC, on average 5-15 points lower than White women (Rubashkin, 2021). Justifiably, the inclusion of the social construct of race came under criticism by scholars as exacerbating racial disparities (Kimani, 2024; Thornton, 2018; Vyas et al., 2019).

Dr Nicholas Rubashkin, an obstetrician from the USA, completed a PhD on the use of race in the VBAC calculator. I am a big fan of Nicholas and his research. We have met a few times and are kindred spirits with our work. His thesis is an essential read. His research is the first time women had been asked about their experience with the VBAC calculator, no qualitative work had been published previously, and the calculator didn't include women or consumer organisations in its design.

Dr Rubashkin interviewed 22 key informants (of the VBAC calculator), 17 clinicians, and 31 women who had a previous caesarean and were either pregnant or recently experienced a subsequent birth. His study found evidence that the VBAC calculator automated racism by systematically giving lower scores to Black and Hispanic women (Rubashkin, 2021).

> *The problem of low scores became not one of accurately communicating statistics, but of managing patient expectations for the greater possibility of failure. The VBAC calculator compounded the decision-making process for women with low scores, many of whom were Black or Hispanic, adding to a challenging situation in*

which many already faced structural vulnerabilities and racism. Black and Hispanic women who were interested in a VBAC more likely faced a dilemma between their commitment to having a VBAC, which itself was a predictive resource, and a low calculator score." Rubashkin, N (2021) page 49.

A new version of the VBAC calculator has now been published, which removes race and replaces it with "chronic hypertension requiring treatment" (yes/no) (Grobman et al., 2021; Thornton, 2023). This new version has been tested on 910 women in the USA, and they found that increased age, history of arrest of dilation or descent for previous caesarean, or chronic hypertension were not associated with VBAC rate (Adjei et al., 2023). The study did find the removal of race produced results that were more consistent with birth outcomes.

Previous Vaginal Birth or VBAC

In the VBAC calculator women, who have a previous VBAC will have a higher VBAC prediction score. This is a factor that makes sense, but I believe has more to do with the woman's brain than her pelvis or uterus.

Historically, an emphasis was placed on the physical dimensions of a woman's pelvis. This stemmed from the belief that a woman's pelvic structure was the primary determinant of whether she could achieve a vaginal birth. This is the old notion of the pelvis being proven.

There was also a concern that successive labours could place increased strain on the uterine scar and increase uterine rupture rates. Mercer et al.'s (2008) research disproved that belief. Mercer et al. (2008) found that VBAC rates increased, and uterine rupture rates decreased, with subsequent VBACs.

Women are so much more than their individual organs or skeletal structures, and vaginal birth has much more to do with the hormonal aspects of environment, safety, comfort, support, and confidence. A woman who has a previous vaginal birth or VBAC has the knowledge that she has had a vaginal birth. She may want to make that experience better, but she has the innate belief that she has birthed a baby through her vagina. That is powerful. Women are powerful.

What clinicians need to do is support women in getting that first vaginal birth as that is the hardest one to get. Subsequent vaginal births become statistically more achievable.

Recurrent Reason for Caesarean Section

The VBAC calculator includes the statement "Indication for prior caesarean of arrest of dilation or descent" (yes/no) and women will score lower if the answer is yes (Grobman et al., 2021).

> *An arrest disorder occurs when, once labor has entered the active phase, dilatation or descent ceases for 2 hours or 1 hour among nulliparas and multiparas, respectively* (Friedman & Cohen, 2023, p. S1106).

This is often diagnosed as a "failure to progress," and often progresses to labour augmentation and the cascade of intervention (Weekend et al., 2024). I explore this in more detail in the active-labour chapter, but suffice to say there is evidence that labour does not always follow an expected progressive pattern, and it can slow and have plateaus, especially towards the end of labour. As a former homebirth midwife, I have personal experience of seeing this.

In Dr Rubashkin's PhD interviews, he found that they didn't always agree with the reason for the previous caesarean to be recurrent, and found they had increased knowledge and understanding about this as they prepared for their next birth (Rubashkin, 2021).

This is supported by my meta-ethnography, which found that women often increased their knowledge following their first caesarean. With this knowledge came a feeling that their previous caesarean was due to iatrogenic factors rather than true "failure to progress" (Keedle et al., 2018b). When we asked women in our national maternity experiences survey what they would do differently next time, the largest category was "Next time I'll be ready," which highlighted the preparation they would do for their next birth.

I am so much more educated since my first birth and can now advocate for myself and educate my husband. The only good thing to come out of my first birth is the strength and passion I now feel surrounding my next birth to be able to fight for myself (ID: 3522) (Keedle et al., 2023, p. 8)

"To just listen and stop quoting guidelines. If a woman wants a VBAC, then support it and don't fear monger.
Also, the language used—failure to progress—is a horrible thing to state. It's 'failure to wait due to guidelines.' Let's take the negativity away and use positive language and ideas on what could enable a VBAC."

Gatekeeping with the VBAC Calculator

The VBAC calculator has unintentionally become a tool used by clinicians to dictate the mode of birth available to women. Rubashkin (2021) found that hospitals used the VBAC calculator score as a gatekeeping tool. For example, if they had a low score then women were actively discouraged from planning a VBAC, supported by documentation so that this was enforced at every health care interaction. Women with high scores had a choice between repeat caesarean and VBAC. In contrast, women with low scores had only one supported choice: a repeat caesarean. A USA survey of midwives found 21.8% used low calculator scores to discourage or prohibit women to plan a VBAC (Thornton et al., 2020).

Women can also feel that the VBAC calculator makes them feel like a failure from the start, and being discouraged from planning a VBAC didn't value the woman's wish to experience labour, regardless of eventual mode of birth (Rubashkin, 2021).

"Treat the mama like she was a healthy pregnant woman about to give birth, not a time bomb about to explode!
Women having VBACs should be informed, but not scared, and have the same opportunities as any pregnant person when in labour."

Summary

In conclusion, I believe the VBAC calculator is not a suitable tool to use with women who are considering their birth-after-caesarean options. Rather than spend time in putting their details into an app to give them an arbitrary probability score, I suggest you spend that time listening to women. What is her previous experience from her perspective? What is her mode of birth preference? Why is that her perspective? In the following chapters, I present a framework that will help you reframe how you support women planning a birth after caesarean.

REFLECTION

Reflect on the information provided in this chapter on the VBAC calculator.

- How has this information informed your thoughts on using the VBAC calculator?
- If you do use the updated calculator, and plan to continue, how are you going to update the information you give women?
- Reflect on a time you have discussed VBAC with a woman, do you know why she wanted to have a VBAC?

CHAPTER 5

How to Support Women to Have Control in Their Birth after Caesarean (BAC)

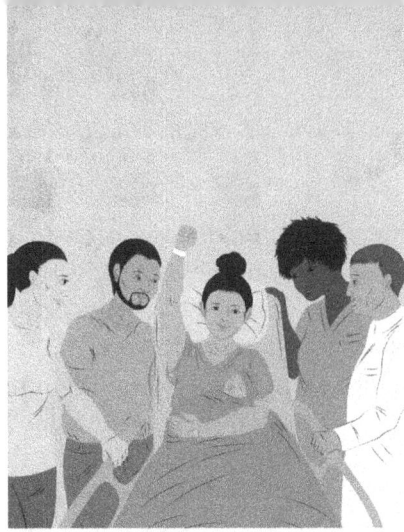

For my PhD, I used sequential mixed methods and started with the qualitative phase. From the meta-ethnography I had undertaken, it was clear that women often had a turbulent journey to have a VBAC. Yet there was limited research focusing in on that journey, certainly not in real-time (Keedle et al., 2018b). The research included in my meta-ethnography had relied on women's recollections of the journey in the postnatal period, or many months or years later. I'm not disputing this style of research, we have relied on it for much of our women's experiences of maternity care research, but for my PhD I wanted to do something different.

I came up with an idea of creating a smartphone application where women could make an audio or video recording immediately following their appointment with their clinician. This led to an education in working with app developers and delight when my idea came to fruition! An app was created that successfully sent recordings from participants phones to a database that I accessed (Keedle et al., 2018a). I recruited 11 women who were currently pregnant and planning a VBAC in Australia. These generous women shared their pregnancy journeys with me, and I ended up with 53 recordings and face-to-face postnatal interviews with all 11. Using narrative analysis, I compared and contrasted the women's stories to look for similarities and differences (Keedle et al., 2019). I had also kept my personal reflections and analysed those too.

One reflection that really stood out for me came after interviewing two women in one day. On paper, they looked so similar, both had planned a VBAC and had a repeat caesarean in labour when they were at full cervical dilation. However, their recollections of their labour and birth experience were vastly different. I'll start with Emma (pseudonym) who was planning a VBAC for her second pregnancy and lived in a regional location. To birth in the local hospital, Emma received her maternity care from a local GP/Obstetrician who attended births. Although he was pleasant, Emma didn't feel that he was supportive of her choice of VBAC. Every appointment he would talk about booking in a repeat caesarean.

When Emma went into labour spontaneously at night, she was able to be mobile at home, and in the morning asked her partner to drop her off at the hospital while he took their child to childcare. In the hospital she was surprised to hear she was fully dilated as the contractions had been manageable and she wasn't feeling an urge to push yet. The doctor told her he would re-examine in 20 minutes. Emma was left on the bed alone as her partner hadn't arrived yet, and still hadn't when the doctor returned and stated she had to have a caesarean as the baby had not descended into her pelvis yet. At her post caesarean debrief, the doctor stated her pelvis wasn't made for birthing. When sharing her birth story with me she said she regretted not engaging with a doula or a midwife and blamed herself for what happened.

In contrast, Arabelle (pseudonym) accessed the midwifery continuity of care program at her closest hospital that supported VBAC, which is called Midwifery Group Practice. She also hired a doula. When her labour started, she travelled to the hospital and during her long labour she was active, upright, used water immersion, and every position out there. After a few hours of being fully dilated, Arabelle could feel that the baby wasn't descending any further. The clinicians caring for her supported her to keep going, but Arabelle made the decision to have a repeat caesarean in labour. On reflection Arabelle reported to me that she felt she had tried absolutely everything during labour, and felt at peace with her decision to have a repeat caesarean.

Although both experiences have similarities, the difference is how the women felt after their experience. Emma felt guilt and regret, Arabelle felt at peace and in control. Neither had a VBAC.

This was one of the many insightful moments during my PhD. I had gone into the PhD thinking it was all about the vagina, or to be more specific, all about pushing a baby out through the vagina, but here were two women who both had a repeat caesarean and felt vastly different about their experiences. I had this lightbulb moment writing up my reflection by the side of the road in my car. It's interesting how we remember where they occurred.

My next insightful moment was during a snowstorm in my hometown in the UK. I had travelled back because my grandmother of 96 years passed away, and I was helping my mum pack up her apartment. Unfortunately, we were then hit with the "beast from the east" snowfall and couldn't drive anywhere. I was able to walk around in the snow though, and found myself escaping into my PhD world in the local library. Up to that point, my analysis had hit a roadblock, and I couldn't see the wood for the trees. In the library, with snow falling outside, I finally got clarity, and the similarities and differences between the stories became clear. After a few scribbles on paper, I could see four trees in the wood, or as they are known, the four factors.

It seems counterintuitive sharing the research process so personally with you, but so many people think research is boring and full of number crunching. It is so much more beautiful than that. It is the inspirational moments, when the jumbled mess of data changes from an indecipherable scribble to a clear diagram. It goes from being a mass of thoughts and ideas, to focusing in on one shining concept. As a mixed-methods researcher, I believe in the value and need for both qualitative and quantitative methodologies. But I do love the magic of qualitative research.

The Four Factors

From 53 recordings and 11 face-to-face interviews. there were four factors that impacted how a woman felt about her planned VBAC, regardless of how she birthed. The factors are having control, having confidence, having a relationship, and staying active in labour. They can be experienced positively or negatively. The culmination of these factors impact whether a woman feels resolved (or other positive feelings) or disappointed (or other negative feelings).

The four factors are on a continuum, and women could feel they experienced a lot or a little of each factor. How a woman experienced the four factors impacted how she felt after the birthing experience. If she felt more in control, had more confidence, had a good relationship with a health care provider, and was more active in labour, the woman would feel more satisfied and resolved. If she felt like she had little control, not much confidence, a poor relationship, and wasn't active in labour, then she would feel disappointed and dissatisfied with her birthing experience.

FIGURE 1: THE FOUR FACTORS (KEEDLE ET AL., 2019)

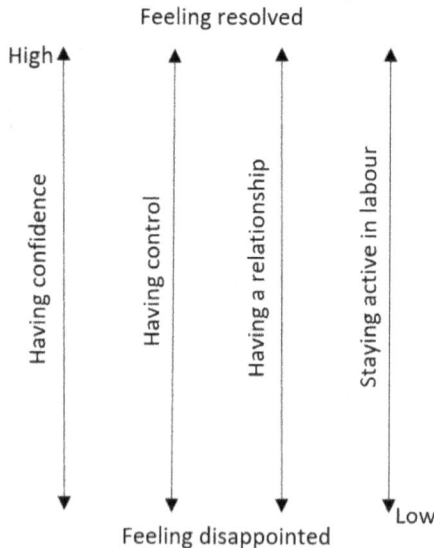

In the third phase of my PhD, I tested the four factors in a national online cross-sectional survey. The survey included purposely written questions and validated survey instruments that covered the four factors. The survey went through face validation using cognitive focus groups. Two papers have been published from the VBAC in Australia (VBAC-AU) survey. One looks at the outcomes across different models of care (Keedle et al., 2020b) and one that analysed the open-text comments in the survey (Keedle et al., 2022).

Since writing my previous book, I have been involved in more research around women's experiences of maternity care and I include the findings in this book. In 2021, our research team led the largest national cross-sectional maternity experiences survey in Australia, the Birth Experience Study (BESt). The co-designed survey included open and closed questions, as well as four validated survey instruments, and resulted in 8,804 completed responses. It is now an international study with more than 14 research groups using the survey in their own countries as part of the Birth Experience Study–International Collaboration (BESt-IC). There have been a range of papers published from the findings, with more in progress. The first publication was a collaboration with a poet who used the open-text comments to create found poetry about birth trauma (Keedle & Willo, 2022). A couple of the poems have been included in this chapter.

The following chapters explore each of the four factors, how clinicians can have a positive impact on each factor, which impacts the overall birthing experience for women. In this chapter, I focus on the first factor: having control.

Having Control

Having control may sound like an unachievable factor since labour and birth is by nature unpredictable. However, this factor includes more than the birth outcome. I describe this factor in one of my PhD papers. Here is an excerpt (Keedle et al., 2019).

> Women who felt that their wishes and choices were respected
> felt more in control of their pregnancy, birthing decisions,

and outcomes ... Feeling in control impacted how Arabelle felt after a repeat emergency caesarean. Arabelle had CoC with a MGP midwife, and went into spontaneous labour after her waters broke at 39 weeks.

My body started pushing, but I still had no urge to push myself, which was kind of weird. But after 4 hours of that I then said it's not going to happen. Like, if it ends up in surgery, I'm completely fine with that. (Arabelle, PN, MGP)

Postnatally, Arabelle reflected on how in control she felt and the benefit of support from a midwife she knew, *"because I think apart from that I was in control the whole way. There was at no point somebody said to me, "No, you can't do that, ... I think the continuity of care, having this same midwife for every single appointment, she stayed with me from the moment I laboured until I went to recovery, and so that made a huge difference"* (Arabelle, PN, MGP)." (Keedle et al., 2019, p. 5).

Supporting Women to Have More Control

So how you can support women to have more control during their entire perinatal journey? In this section, I present three ways you can support women: by exploring their previous birth experience, enabling the use of birth plans and using respectful language.

Exploring the Previous Birth Experience

Every woman who has a previous caesarean has a story about her birthing experience. For many that story will be traumatic, and may well include a loss of control of the experience they were hoping for. To support women in their next birth experience, we need to give women the opportunity to talk about their previous birth. Through listening, you will invariably hear about difficult situations and how you react in those situations will have a significant impact on whether the woman feels you are supportive, or not.

Addressing Birth Trauma

In the VBAC-AU survey, we found that two thirds of women reported their previous birth was traumatic (Keedle et al., 2020b). This is double the birth trauma rate found in previously published papers that include vaginal and caesarean births. In BESt, there was a reported birth trauma rate of 28% (Keedle & Dahlen, 2023).

FIGURE 2: *MOTHER GUILT*, POEM BY PIXIE WILLO

Mother Guilt

By the time I reached the pushing stage, I ... was coached to hold my breath ... and pushing mid contraction ... I had a time limit ... the baby had to be out within the hour... Eventually, the doctor said ... the vacuum is ... our best option ... for proceeding ... which filled my heart with dread ... I did not have time to answer... or consider my options as ... Baby at an angle ... putting pressure on my hips ... caused ... a painful contraction ... Without consent, the doctor... ... began the vacuum process ... It felt like a hundred strangers ... had swarmed into the room ... all here for the freak show ... My screaming continued ... my partner crying as ... he watched on helplessly ... They moved onto forceps ... I was yelling to my partner... *"This is wrong!"*... *"This is wrong!"*... Everything about this was wrong ... The pain ... At one point ... was ... Unbearable ... I thought I was dying ... I just needed ... a break ... to ... catch my breath ... so ... I started yelling ... *"Stop! Stop! Please stop!"*... My cries ignored ... they did not stop ... they did not pause ... When my baby came out ... her fraught cries ... like mine ... like ... she was in agony ... That will haunt me forever ... my first words to her ... were ... sorry ... for how wrong it all was ... how she deserved better ... how I had failed ... to protect her... in the jaws ... of a ... Humanless system...

(Keedle & Willo, 2022, p. 3)

REFLECTION

Reflect on the poem *Mother Guilt*.

- Reading it out loud, what does the rhythm remind you of?
- How does the poem make you feel?
- How do you think the woman would feel after this birthing experience?

There are a variety of definitions around birth trauma. I firmly believe in Cheryl Beck's position that birth trauma is in the "eye of the beholder," making the identification of birth trauma with the woman (Beck, 2004).

I also believe that birth trauma is an umbrella term that encompasses different experiences. Under the umbrella (Figure 3), is lack of support, loss of control, fearing for the baby's life or their own life, and physical trauma, such as perineal tears, episiotomy, and caesarean wounds. Also under the umbrella is obstetric violence and racism. The use of the word "birth" is potentially misleading as the trauma can occur at any or a multitude of times throughout the perinatal period. Maybe the term "perinatal trauma" would be more suitable.

FIGURE 3: BIRTH/PERINATAL TRAUMA UMBRELLA

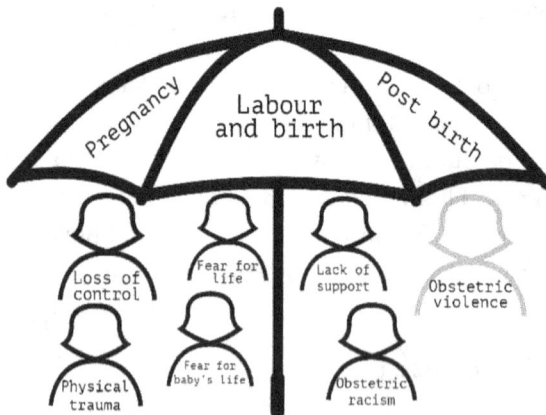

As clinicians it is important to recognise the individuality of birth trauma. One woman may experience one or more of the events under the umbrella and not feel traumatised, yet another woman will. Let's have a look at each type of trauma under the umbrella. I recognise this isn't an exhaustive list, but it does include what comes up most frequently in research.

Loss of Control

As mentioned earlier, having control is related to how in control the woman feels she was regarding her wishes, decisions, and outcomes. Loss of control is integrated in feeling the birth was a traumatic experience. A meta-analysis and concept analysis of 44 studies defined a loss of control related to birth trauma as:

> *Women feel deprived of decision-making and informed consent, their birth process is completely in the hands of care providers, and reality is not moving toward their expectations, which makes them feel out of control* (Sun et al., 2023, p. 4).

In my narrative analysis paper we shared the story of Carley and how she felt out of control(Keedle et al., 2019). Here is an excerpt from the paper:

> Once Carley knew her planned homebirth after caesarean (HBAC) was going to be a planned induction of labour in hospital, she *"just cried the whole Sunday"* (Carley, PN, PPM) because *"I knew if I was being induced, that was it, it was not going to work"* (Carley, PN, PPM). Carley had a Foley catheter inserted to induce labour overnight, and the next day had her membranes ruptured. When labour didn't "progress," she requested synthetic oxytocin but was refused by the obstetric team. When reflecting on how she was treated in labour she felt that by not being given options she was denied control of her situation.

> *"You need to give people choices. You need to give people options. And we weren't, at any point in that whole scene, we were not near a situation where you would, you know, an emergency that overrules everything"* (Carley, PN, PPM)" (Keedle et al., 2019, p. 6).

It is a long journey for women to develop resilience and understanding after feeling a loss of control after a traumatic birth. Not all women have the support to make that journey. A qualitative study from the UK described how women used their faith, the experience of motherhood, support from family and friends, and self-care to gain a renewed strength and take back control of their life (Brown et al., 2022).

The words "renewed strength" reminded me of a woman I had the honour to support as a midwife. Her first birth resulted in a forceps birth with a bilateral episiotomy. When she showed me her baby photos, I was shocked. The baby looked so battered and bruised. The couple described how other parents would look judgementally at them when they walked into the special care nursery, perhaps thinking they had harmed their baby.

During her next pregnancy, she joined a woman's group I had set up in a regional area of New South Wales, and she was getting antenatal care from a different hospital from the first. As her pregnancy progressed, she was beginning to experience similar red flags as last time due to having gestational diabetes that she was managing well with diet and exercise. At the end of her pregnancy her stress was increasing (as was mine as the observer), and I offered to support her in the hospital during labour and birth. After that offer she went into labour that night. I met her at the hospital, and we were fortunate that a dear colleague midwife of mine was in labour ward, and her student midwife was also in attendance.

As we walked into the room, carrying the vision board she had created, we saw how the student midwife had prepared the room. Low lighting, battery operated tea light candles, soft music, and printed affirmations on the walls. After a few hours she birthed her baby on the mattress on the floor on all fours, her head being supported by her seated husband. She listened to my quiet voice. She birthed her baby by lowering her body and the baby gently slipped onto the mattress. No one touching her or the baby at all. All I had to say was, "you can pick up your baby now." She looked transformed! She had delayed cord clamping, an intact perineum, and skin to skin for a few hours.

Postnatally, I saw this woman become so strong and confident that I mentioned it to her. She replied by saying she had regained the strength and confidence that had been taken from her in the first birth and now felt stronger than ever. We have such responsibility in our hands. We can tear women down or support them to tap into their own strength and power.

Fear for Own or Baby's Life

In birth trauma research many women and partners identify experiencing a fear for their own (or partners) or their baby's life during their traumatic birthing experience (Keedle et al., 2015; Shorey & Wong, 2022; Sun et al., 2023). This may be a real or a perceived fear, or a fear exaggerated by clinicians. In a meta-synthesis of 19 studies on traumatic birth, Shorey and Wong (2022) found ten of 19 studies examined the profound fear experienced by women and their partners during childbirth, with a primary focus on concerns for maternal and foetal safety. Women's fears centred on potential harm to their babies, including birth complications, neonatal mortality, and the recurrence of previous traumatic birth experiences. Some women described near-death experiences, with vivid recollections of out-of-body sensations and a sense of impending doom. These experiences were often compounded by perceived incompetence from health care providers and inadequate resources in certain settings.

Partners reported intense fear of losing their partners and children during childbirth. They also expressed significant distress at witnessing their partner's physical and emotional suffering while feeling powerless to intervene. There is a close link with feeling a loss of control. This sense of powerlessness was a major contributor to their overall fear and anxiety, particularly when their own lives or the lives of their babies felt threatened (Shorey & Wong, 2022).

Lack of Support

Women describe feelings of neglect, avoidance by staff, and a general lack of support when they were describing their traumatic birth experience (Shorey & Wong, 2022). A lack of support can either be from personal support, such as partners, family or friends, or professional clinician support. The lack of support can start during the pregnancy, for example a family member who doesn't support the woman choosing a VBAC (Keedle et al., 2015).

Support during labour has significant benefits. A Cochrane systematic review found continuous support during labour increased spontaneous vaginal birth, decreased time of labour, decreased caesareans, instrumental births, use of analgesia (including epidurals), and low five-minute Apgar scores, alongside decreasing negative feelings about birth (Bohren et al., 2017).

I do understand that many women are unable to receive that kind of continuous support from clinicians due to time restraints, lack of staffing and resources, and busy workloads. This is where it is essential that doulas are included in the support team.

A scoping review on the effect of doulas suggests that doula support during the perinatal period may have significant positive impacts on maternal and neonatal outcomes (Sobczak et al., 2023). The included studies indicated a potential association between doula guidance and reduced rates of caesarean section and preterm birth, and shortened labour duration. The emotional support provided by doulas appears to effectively alleviate maternal anxiety and stress during pregnancy and childbirth. Doula support, particularly among low-income women, has been shown to improve breastfeeding initiation and duration, with benefits, such as quicker lactogenesis II onset. These findings suggest that doulas can be a valuable resource for birthing mothers. This review raises important questions regarding equitable access to doula services, and the potential role of doula support in improving health outcomes for women across all socioeconomic levels (Sobczak et al., 2023).

Physical Trauma

As mentioned in Chapter 3, women who have severe perineal trauma following a birth may experience mental health issues in the postnatal period (Molyneux et al., 2024; Opondo et al., 2023).

A UK study of 4,578 women by Opondo et al. (2023) investigated the association between perineal trauma and subsequent psychological outcomes in women. Findings revealed a strong link between perineal trauma and increased physical symptoms postpartum. Notably, the severity of physical symptoms significantly predicted the likelihood of experiencing depression, anxiety, and posttraumatic stress disorder (PTSD) symptoms. While a direct association between perineal trauma and PTSD was observed, no direct link was found between trauma and depression or anxiety. These findings highlight the crucial role of effective assessment and management of physical symptoms in the post-partum period to minimise both physical and psychological morbidity for women.

There is limited research on the psychological impact of caesarean wound complications however this qualitative study from the UK sheds some light on this issue. This study by Djatmika et al. (2024) explored the lived experiences of women with slow-to-heal caesarean section wounds. Utilising Interpretative Phenomenological Analysis, key themes emerged: 1) the intertwined nature of physical and emotional healing, 2) the challenges of balancing caregiving responsibilities with the demands of their own recovery, and 3) the process of adapting to a "new normal" shaped by the prolonged healing process. Findings highlighted the impact of delayed wound healing on women's sense of agency, their ability to fulfil their maternal roles, and their overall well-being. These findings emphasised the need for a holistic approach to understanding and addressing the complexities of caesarean birth recovery, particularly for women experiencing delayed wound healing. This research underscores the importance of recognising and address-ing the often "invisible" challenges faced by these women.

Obstetric Racism

Obstetric racism refers to the systemic racism within the health care system that results in disparities in the reproductive health care experi-ences of Black, Indigenous or People of Colour (Aseffa et al., 2024; Davis, 2019; Macedo et al., 2020; Rubashkin et al., 2024; Williamson, 2021), and is a major factor in experiencing a traumatic birth (Dmowska et al.,

2023). This includes the historical and contemporary legacies of slavery, eugenics, and other forms of racial discrimination that have shaped health care for Black, Indigenous or People of Colour (Owens, 2017).

Obstetric racism manifests in various ways, such as medical neglect, dehumanising treatment, lack of respect for autonomy, and disparities in access to quality health care. For example, Black and First Nations women are more likely to experience preterm birth, low birth weight, and maternal mortality compared to White women (Brown et al., 2021; Davis, 2020; Lawton et al., 2021). These disparities are rooted in systemic racism that permeates the health care system. Recognising and address-ing obstetric racism is crucial for improving maternal and child health outcomes for Black, Indigenous or People of Colour and requires a commitment to dismantling systemic barriers, and ensuring equitable access to quality health care for all.

Obstetric Violence

Following my caesarean for my first baby, I remember the obstetrician visiting me in the postnatal ward and telling me I was a good candidate for a VBAC for my next birth. She continued to explain that she had performed a vaginal examination on me when I was on the operating table with a spinal anaesthetic on board, and I was already 8 cm with my breech baby. After she left the room, I felt uncomfortable and I wasn't sure why. That was good news right? It took a while for me to realise that was an internal vaginal examination done **without my consent.** I had no knowledge at all until she told me about it. Years later, I found the words that described what had happened to me: obstetric violence (OV).

Fifteen years later, I was writing a paper on Australian women's experiences of obstetric violence from our BESt dataset (Keedle et al., 2024). It was the first paper identifying that obstetric violence existed in Australia, and found that more than one in 10 women experienced obstetric violence that left them feeling dehumanised, powerless, and violated. The violations included physical assaults, episiotomies done without consent, and vaginal examinations described as sexual assaults.

Obstetric violence has been recognised as a form of gendered violence by a Special Rapporteur to the United Nations (Simonovic, 2019), the European Union (Quattrocchi, 2024) and the International Confederation of Midwives (International Confederation of Midwives, 2024). The violence can be perpetuated by any clinician, midwife, nurse, doctor, radiologist, etc and is often exacerbated by patriarchal systemic institutions.

For clinicians, the issue of OV can feel insurmountable and an issue for others to address, alongside feeling like a personal attack since most clinicians don't go into their careers to cause harm. That's the tricky issue of OV: it can be veiled behind routine policies and practices that you do every day. One example of that is vaginal examinations. These have become a routine practice in labour, and some clinicians perform them during pregnancy. Routine vaginal examinations are not evidence-based. A Cochrane systematic review found no improvement in maternity or neonatal outcomes with routine vaginal examinations (Moncrieff et al., 2022). As I describe in this excerpt of our OV paper, the way vaginal examinations (VE) are performed is completely in the powerful hands of the clinician.

A negative VE experience can be exacerbated by the power imbalance between HCP and women. With the woman lying supine, her legs are opened and gloved hands insert two fingers into the vagina to check cervical dilation and the presenting part of the baby. The VE can be quick or long, easy or complex, gentle or rough, and this is all dependent on the HCP. If you add a lack of consent and explanation, it is easy to see how this practice could be experienced as a violent, intimate assault (Keedle et al., 2024, p. 18).

I understand that the use of vaginal examinations is not going to magically disappear, and not have a role in labour care, but I do think there are small changes that clinicians can implement before each and every examination using trauma-informed care principles. Let's have a look at what the principles are first.

Obstetric violence is a harmful aspect of birth trauma. It destroys the trust between women and clinicians. Women are often silenced and gaslighted following an experience of OV by the very institutions and clinicians that should have provided respectful maternity care. It's never okay.

FIGURE 4: *OBSTETRIC VIOLENCE* BY PIXIE WILLO

The Dr entered the room
the sight of him caused
me to burst into tears
everything became
A terrifying blur
He
Awakened my fears
He
brutally took away all control
my plan not respected
completely shattering my world,
my innate intuition.
Completely ignored.
He
put his fingers inside me
Without
My
Consent
I don't believe I consented
scared and vulnerable
Scared for my baby
they pulled me from the water,
Nobody heard
The words I was screaming
from the very beginning
Nobody heard

(Keedle & Willo, 2022, p. 4)

Trauma-Informed Care

A Trauma-Informed Care (TIC) framework is crucial in maternity settings as I have presented the high prevalence of trauma among women, and the potential for the birthing experience itself to be re-traumatising.

Trauma-Informed Care recognises that many women have experienced trauma in their lives, such as childhood abuse, violence, sexual assault, or other adverse events, including birth trauma. These experiences can significantly impact their mental and physical health, influencing their responses to pregnancy, childbirth, and postpartum experiences (NSW Health, 2023). By incorporating Trauma-Informed Care principles, clinicians can create a safer and more supportive environment for women, minimising the risk of re-traumatisation during their care.

Trauma-Informed Care principles, from the NSW Health Integrated Trauma-Informed Care Framework (NSW Health, 2023)include:

- Safety
- Trustworthiness
- Collaboration
- Choice
- Integration
- Empowerment
- Culture, gender history and identity

Returning to vaginal examinations, let's explore how can they be performed using trauma-informed principles. The first step is information giving in a respectful way to assist women to have **choice** in the procedure. One way of doing that is using the BRAIN acronym.

- **B:** Benefits - What are the benefits of this decision for you and your baby?
- **R:** Risks - What are the risks of this decision for you and your baby?
- **A:** Alternatives - Are there other options?
- **I:** Intuition - What do you feel is right and safe for you?
- **N:** Nothing - What happens if you do nothing?

This tool is a great method to ensure you have covered the risks and benefits of the procedure, the alternatives of not having an examination and what could happen with that. Offer her the **choice** over where the procedure will take place (e.g., in the birthing pool if she is utilising that, leaning back on an easy chair, on the birthing mat on the floor or on the bed. If possible, give her the **choice** on who will do the examination). She may wish for a provider she knows, or a woman. You should be confident and competent to do a vaginal examination in different positions. Give her control and **choice** on the language she can use to stop the procedure at any time, and show **trustworthiness** by respecting this. Finally, you can ask the women to express how she is feeling right now.

It is also important to consider the position of your body when you are giving this information. Many women will be on the bed during this conversation. Where are you? Are you standing and towering over her, are you sitting on the bed, or are you sitting on a chair beside her. Remember the power differential. Standing over the woman reinforces that power differential and may impact her ability to advocate for herself. Sitting on the bed may be problematic if the woman has experienced any trauma on a bed, such as childhood sexual trauma or sexual assault. The woman has limited safe space around her when you sit on her bed, and this can increase the power differential. Sitting on a chair beside the bed, especially if you are lower or at the same level as her head, and there is space between yourself and the woman, is potentially a trauma-informed approach.

If the woman gives informed consent to the procedure, ask how you can make the procedure **safe** for her. "I would like you to consider how I can make this procedure **safe** for you?" Then give her space without you there to consider that. Leave the room to give her a breather. On your return, ask if she has any thoughts on this and then show respect and **trustworthiness** by supporting her wishes. She may ask for a support person, or that she can listen to music, or that you tell her what you are doing and feeling throughout. There are many suggestions she may come up with, and they may or may not be connected to remaining in control following a previous traumatic experience. Also remember that you don't need to know about her previous traumatic experiences. It is her decision to share with your or not, not your right to know.

During the procedure, if she asks you to stop, then stop. You don't continue because you don't have all the information that you need. You stop. After the procedure wait for her to no longer be exposed and then sit back in that chair to discuss the procedure and what you felt and how this impacts her labour.

This may seem like an idealistic and time-consuming practice, but it is a way that you can address obstetric violence at an individual level. However, it is even greater than that. You have impacted her experience of maternity care and given her power back. You have potentially impacted another clinician in the room who has witnessed you perform a trauma-informed vaginal examination. They may ask you about it or start using the techniques that you did. Your one practice change can have a ripple effect throughout your maternity department. Never underestimate the power of positive change.

REFLECTION

Reflect on performing vaginal examinations

- How do you feel after reading the section about obstetric violence and vaginal examinations? Angry, sad, frustrated, indifferent?

- After reading my suggested trauma informed way of performing vaginal examinations, do you think you could incorporate that into your practice?

- If a student or clinician witnessed you perform a trauma-informed vaginal examination, how would you talk about why you did it that way?

- Reflect on the first and subsequent times you did this. How did it feel for you and the woman?

- Reflect on the woman's responses to how to make the procedure safe for them. Were there any surprising suggestions or ones that made you think?

- Consider getting feedback from women on how they felt about the trauma-informed vaginal examination.

Secondary Traumatic Stress

Within the concept of safety it is vital to consider the wellbeing of clinicians who witness birth trauma and other traumatic events, as these can lead to secondary traumatic stress (Bayri Bingol et al., 2021; Kendall-Tackett & Beck, 2022; Leinweber et al., 2017). As a clinician you need to recognise when you are requiring extra support and strategies to assist in your healing and recovery following secondary traumatic stress and/or burnout. Sometimes it is the people around you that see the impact. Those conversations may be difficult, but can be healing. Recovery is achievable, and you deserve to experience that.

There are resources available for clinicians and I suggest you investigate what support you can access in your area. One important resource in Australia is the Nurse and Midwife Support website and helpline: https://www.nmsupport.org.au

Ongoing Impact of Birth Trauma

For some women who have experienced a traumatic birth, they may experience mental health issues, such as anxiety, depression, and post-traumatic stress disorders (Ertan et al., 2021). Studies have also found experiencing birth trauma can lead to women demonstrating increased anxiety around their baby's health and their parenting abilities (Molloy et al., 2021; Priddis et al., 2018).

Birth Debriefing

Recognising that up to two thirds of women with a previous caesarean may have experienced birth trauma, how are you going to approach this during their next pregnancy? The first step is to offer the woman the opportunity to talk about their previous birth, and for you to actively listen. This isn't the opportunity to defend or argue with them about their perspective of what happened, but to listen with the intent to understand how they feel about the experience.

In BESt, we asked women about their experience with birth debriefing (Bannister et al, 2025). The key findings included a high demand for debriefing among women, with many expressing a desire to discuss their birth experiences. Women who participated in debriefing generally found it helpful, valuing the opportunity to process emotions, address trauma, and gain closure. Importantly, women emphasised the need for woman-centred debriefing, prioritising their individual needs and preferences.

Debriefing can serve as an early intervention for addressing potential psychological distress following childbirth. However, current evidence on the effectiveness of debriefing is limited due to variations in its definition, implementation, and evaluation methods (Thomson et al., 2021).

Key recommendations include offering debriefing to all women, prioritising woman-centred care, providing multiple opportunities for debriefing, involving appropriately trained health care providers with the time to sit with women, and conducting further research to investigate the most effective models of debriefing and to evaluate its impact on maternal mental health outcomes.

In the meantime, consider how you discuss women's previous birth experiences and give women the time to tell you how they feel about it and what they would like to do differently next time.

"Listen and ask the woman why she wants a certain birth. What it means to her and why it's important. Ask her how many children she wants. Be clear, open, and transparent in a compassionate way. Be supportive and understanding, and actually help the women achieve the birth she wants. Learn all you can to support the woman to have that birth. If you don't have confidence in her choice, research it so you understand why you don't have confidence. Could it be bias? Lack of understanding? Clash of birth values? If you can't support a woman in that capacity, match her with someone who will give her the best chance."

Birth Plans

The concept of birth plans was pioneered by childbirth educators and anthropologists Sheila Kitzinger in the UK and Penny Simkin in the USA in the early 1980s (Kitzinger, 1992, 2015). Intended to foster trust and cooperation between women and health care providers, birth plans were envisioned as a tool for communication and shared decision-making during pregnancy and labour (Kitzinger, 1992; Leap & Hunter, 2016). Modern birth plans vary in format, from simple checklists to customisable online templates. The World Health Organization recognizes the potential benefits of birth plans in improving maternal and newborn health (WHO, 2009).

In my PhD research, 75% of women who had experienced VBAC reported creating a birth plan (Keedle et al., 2020a). Notably, women receiving midwifery continuity of care were significantly more likely to report their clinicians supported their birth plans compared to those receiving continuity of care with doctors or receiving standard antenatal care. This highlights the importance of provider support in the birth planning process. From a midwifery perspective, I believe that creating a birth plan can empower women by facilitating open communication with their clinicians and fostering a sense of control over their birth experience, regardless of how the actual birth unfolds.

An integrative review of 11 studies by Bell et al. (2022) focused on the purpose and process for birth plans. The findings suggest that collaborative birth plan creation, involving open communication and shared decision-making between women and their care providers, leads to more positive outcomes, including improved communication, increased satisfaction, and a greater sense of control for women. Challenges include inconsistent implementation, limited access to comprehensive antenatal education, and power imbalances within the health care system. The review emphasises the importance of shifting from a focus on the document itself to a focus on the process of collaborative planning and communication between women and their health care providers. A universal, consistent, and woman-centred approach to birth-plan creation is recommended, focusing on open communication, shared decision-making, and addressing individual needs and preferences.

There are a variety of ways you can encourage and incorporate birth plans into your practice. You can explore the use of a "Birth Map" (Bell et al., 2023), or even use the art therapy method that I describe in my previous book (Keedle, 2022) as two examples. I do think it is important to consider your own biases. Complete the reflection below to explore this.

REFLECTION

Reflect on the use of birth plans.

- If you were to develop a birth plan, what would it look like? What are your preferences? What's important to you?

- How do you imagine your ideal labour and birth? If you were to draw this what would be there? What environment are you birthing in? Who is there? What are you using in labour to help with the challenging waves of contractions? What's your birthing position?

- If you were to think about the worst outcomes for your birth, what would it look like to you?

- Imagine you are caring for a woman whose birth plan is very different than yours, with a different mode of birth, location, pain relief choices, support people, the works. How do you think your care may be impacted due to this difference? Recognising this can help you address your biases.

- Imagine you are caring for a woman who says she had a traumatic birth, and you were involved in the birth. What advice would you give her? How would you validate her feelings without taking it personally?

- What support services are you aware of for yourself and your colleagues if you have witnessed a traumatic birth?

Respectful Language

The final aspect of supporting women to have control is to use respectful language. This may sound obvious, but in my PhD VBAC study 51% of women had received hurtful comments from clinicians (Keedle et al., 2020a). In a content analysis of all the qualitative comments women submitted in the survey there were many comments that were coercive in nature (Keedle et al., 2022). One example of this coercive language is in the quote below:

> *"One obstetrician I saw at 20 weeks said "if you try for a VBAC, your husband will end up with a dead wife, a dead baby, and a toddler to raise on his own." I have obviously refused to see him again and have booked all future hospital appointments with a VBAC-supportive OB" (CP161, Public hospital care).* (Keedle et al., 2022, p. 8)

Women can also be subjected to body shaming, and as discussed earlier, obstetric racism. Woman you care for want their babies to be born alive. Therefore, using the "dead-baby card" (when a clinician states the baby will die if the woman does or doesn't do an action) so that the woman is guilted into changing her preference to suit your own level of comfort is never okay. Every woman deserves respectful maternity care and that includes being communicated with respectfully.

Summary

This chapter has explored some big issues, and you may be full of uncomfortable feelings and memories. They are vitally important issues that need to be addressed. Understanding what women have experienced is a step towards preventing future trauma. To support women to have more control we need to understand how they lost that control in previous births.

"Work out whether the previous C-section was planned or unplanned, and whether it was traumatic. Ask and listen as to why was it traumatic. Perhaps in that conversation, they realise it was traumatic so having on hand details of local perinatal mental health services (i.e., counselling, psychs, etc). Ask what they want to be different and what they want to know. Remove myths and fear-based dialogue around VBAC. Have convo about repeat C-section and one or two things that would make it better. Write that down, then leave the conversation there and focus on preparing for a VBAC. Storytelling is powerful so having a few podcast episodes of successful VBACs, as well as unrealised yet empowering C-sections. Remind them that policy is advice or guidelines, not law."

CHAPTER 6

How to Support Women to Have Increased Confidence in Their BAC

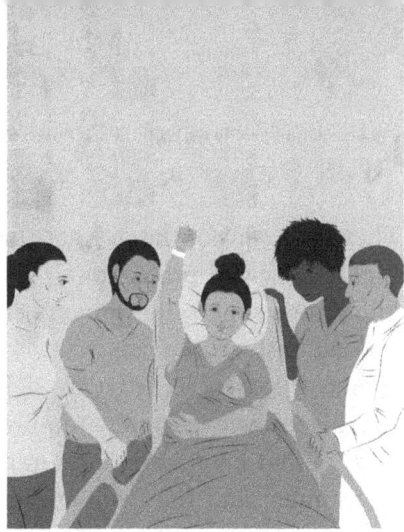

This chapter explores how to support women as they increase their confidence in their ability to have a VBAC. The main focus is on how women need providers to increase their own confidence in BAC. In the VBAC-AU survey, we asked women if they felt their clinician was confident in the woman's ability to have a VBAC, both during pregnancy and during labour. Seventy-two percent of women felt their clinician was confident in their ability to have a VBAC during pregnancy, but it dropped to 68% during labour. What this shows is that women are perceptive to how confident they feel you are about their ability to have a VBAC. This is important to women. When a woman is planning a VBAC she wants to know that you believe she can do it.

Knowledge is Power–Encourage It!

An aspect of patriarchy in medical philosophy has been the hegemonic belief in authoritative knowledge. Introduced by feminists Oakley (Oakley, 1993), Jordan (Jordan, 1997) and Davis-Floyd (Davis-Floyd, 1993), the technocratic model of birth is that obstetricians hold the authoritative knowledge on all aspects of perinatal care and they pass it down to other professionals on the hierarchical ladder. This is the "doctor knows best" belief which can lead to a "God Complex." The result is that women either feel that they are not experts on their body, or they are discredited by the recognised experts when they do try to speak out.

There is a tension here. I get that. There is certainly knowledge that highly educated professionals hold that others may not, but does that knowledge supersede women's choices or her instincts? I don't believe it does. Instead, we can actively understand that the woman has the right to make choices that are right for her. Our role is to support her by sharing knowledge as she requires or asks for it. The midwifery philosophy is that pregnancy, labour, and birth are physiological life events for women, and that women benefit from being in partnership with a midwife (Dixon et al., 2023). I think other health care professionals can benefit from that philosophy too. Our main role in pregnancy is in the realm of primary health care and public health. We listen, provide support and education, offer screening, and at times, we provide treatment. I think we could increase our skills in providing health education, especially how we communicate that with women.

Don't underestimate the ability to source knowledge as a consumer. Back when I was a paediatric nurse, I knew the parent of a child with a chronic illness or disability were often the most acquainted with the research, treatments, and individual requirements of their child's medical issues. I learnt so much when I was working alongside these parents for 12 hours in intensive care. At the first sign of anything, I would turn to the parent and say, "is this okay for them?" Together we could intervene early. As a mum, I've navigated the world of neurodiversity for my children, so I have some insight into the knowledge required to advocate.

We are fortunate to live in the age of the internet and can access information at the tap of our fingers on a smart phone. I sense a shiver going down your spine. Does the thought of Dr. Google give you chills? Have you heard, or even said these words to women, *"Don't Google it, though"*? Let's explore this a bit further. What message are you giving when you say to someone to not look something up on Google?

You may think you are protecting them from misinformation; that they won't be able to tell the difference between evidence-based information and the many ludicrous claims online. Nope, that's not what you're doing. What you are doing is slamming a door of open communication in their face, like a tempestuous teenager who has been asked to clean the kitchen. What do you think will happen? Whatever you have suggested not to be Googled will be Googled by the time she leaves the clinic. She will continue to Google it and learn some evidence-based information and maybe some dubious information. She may have a bit of confusion over the information, but you have already closed that door of communication, so she is unable to discuss it with you at the next appointment. To do this she would need to admit to disobeying you and subject herself to shame and disapproval. What if she followed the incorrect advice? I guess you are not to blame as you didn't tell her do it. But you didn't educate her either.

Another way to handle this is to understand that we are curious creatures. We naturally seek knowledge from the easiest methods, and for most of us that will be the internet. It's better to acknowledge that and open the door of communication.

You could say, "So at the next appointment, we recommend you have screening for [insert issue]. I'm sure you would like to learn more about it before the screening, I can recommend some good websites to you that have evidence-based information. Have a look at [insert good websites]. You may find other information on it online too and that can be helpful. If any of the information is different from the info given on the websites I have suggested, please make a note of the websites and we can look at the pages together at your next appointment." This creates an open door to information seeking and sharing. You will play a vital role in how to distinguish between reputable evidence-based information and potentially harmful information online. You may also learn something. Identifying evidence-based information online is a vital skill that we could all learn more of.

> "I am in the midst of this at the moment; 37+4 planning a HBAC. The best thing my midwife has done for me is shown what total confidence she has in me and my body. Reminding me that I CAN do this. She also created a client portal with a whole heap of handy VBAC-related content, which was highly useful."

> **REFLECTION** 💬
>
> Build up your resource of reliable online evidence-based information.
>
> - How are you certain this is evidence-based information?
> - Is it written in consumer-friendly language?
> - Are they accessible to all?
> - Are they available in low literacy or different languages?
> - How up to date is the information?
> - How will you share the website? – Do you have a link to online resources on your website or a written list you can give women?
> - Make sure you check the links are still working before you direct people to them.

Why Vaginal Birth is Important to Women

- Do you believe in the value of vaginal birth?
- Do you think vaginal birth is natural?
- Do you think having a vaginal birth can be healing or empowering for women?

I think it can be hard to be positive and continue believing in the value of vaginal birth when working in the current maternity system. After all, it has become so rare to see women have spontaneous, intervention- and drug-free vaginal births. Those rare events tend to happen in hospitals at night, or within continuity of care midwifery models, or at home. A morning shift in a birthing ward is full of women having their inductions of labour started. Strap in for the cascade of interventions!

What is the rhetoric of birth in your mind? Do you feel it is inherently risky? Do you feel you can trust women to birth vaginally? Do you believe women want the interventions and don't care about the mode of birth?

In the moments of labour, birth, and the postnatal period in hospital it may be easy to think this. A woman may smile and say thank you when you offer interventions or pain relief. She may smile and say thank you when you explain why she had a caesarean. But then she goes home, and sometime later, reflects on her experience.

This is where we have seen insights in the BESt survey. We asked the question, "Would you do anything different if you were to have another baby?", and 6,101 women responded (Keedle et al., 2023). It was an interesting question as we gave women the option to wave a magic wand and think about what they would want in their ideal birth. In summary, there were four categories of comments. The biggest category was "Next time I'll be ready," where women highlighted how they would get better prepared through educating and avoiding intervention.

> *Yes, instead of trusting the care provider to provide me with the latest evidence-based research I will research for it myself and arm myself with it so that I get the care I deserve. I feel my best chances of VBAC is to be prepared both educationally and emotionally. I will never trust a care provider as much as I did with my first pregnancy. My maternal instincts will always come first* (ID: 2952) (Keedle et al., 2023, p. 8).

The second biggest category was "I want a specific birth experience." In this category of 2,872 comments, 60% stated the wish for a vaginal birth, 16% focused on wanting to be upright and active during labour, and 8% were about birth environment. Fifteen percent of comments were women wanting a caesarean for their next birth.

I think this shows that women often feel that clinicians deceived them once they reflect on the birthing experience. When you are seeing the smiles and hearing the "thank you," they might not have had time to process what happened.

Let's focus in on what women with a previous caesarean say about vaginal birth. In the VBAC-AU survey, we asked the open text question:

"Why was planning a VBAC important to you?" There were 258 responses that were coded into 330 items of coding using content analysis.

The largest category was "To experience birth," and consisted of comments that highlighted the desire to go through the physiological birthing process. Out of the 85 items of coding, 34 used the term "natural" such as: *"Because vaginal birth is the natural way for childbirth all being well with mother and baby."* Table 3 lists the different categories and gives an exemplar for each category. This data hasn't been published in a journal article, so you are seeing it here first!

TABLE 3: REASONS FOR PLANNING A VBAC

Category	Items of coding	Exemplar
To experience birth	85	I don't want to miss out on one of the most amazing things that a woman is made to do. I want to take back my control, which I didn't have with the birth of my son.
Better Recovery	76	Because it is better for my baby and a better experience/recovery for me.
Lower risks	46	Better for baby and my own health, short and long term.
Avoiding surgery/ intervention	40	Because why would you have major surgery if you could avoid it?
Empowerment	33	Also very important is the physiological hormonal response that is just the most amazing thing in the entire world. It sets the mother (me) up to feel amazing and empowered, and to be able to form a strong attachment to my baby and get through the coming months of sleeplessness with grace.
Traumatic caesarean	28	To heal emotionally from the trauma of the c-sections I've had.
Improve bonding / breastfeeding	18	To promote the best possible start to my breastfeeding journey. Last time took a few days to establish.
Better options for future births	4	To have more children and be able to care for a toddler with a newborn.
Total comments	330	

Vaginal birth matters to women: fact, based on evidence. This doesn't buy into the "vaginal birth is good and caesarean is bad" rhetoric though. The use of a caesarean is necessary in certain situations, but it is a surgical procedure compared to a vaginal birth.

There are many consumer organisations that want to fight against the "normal" vaginal birth movement and blame the promotion of normal vaginal birth as damaging. There are many women who feel offended by the term "normal vaginal birth." I think that is problematic. We need to hold vaginal birth as sacred. That should be the goal, if that is what the woman wants. If though, for myriad reasons, a vaginal birth is no longer possible, it is vital that the woman can have a gentle, respectful caesarean, and not feel that she was a failure.

Believe I am capable of a VBAC!

Find the 'Why' in Women's Stories

One way you can increase your confidence in VBAC is connecting with women's stories of their VBAC. There are many ways you can do this. Here are two.

1. Read a book. –In my first book, *Birth after Caesarean, Your Journey to a Better Birth,* I include 15 stories from women who had a VBAC with extra challenges.

2. Listen to podcasts.–We have great podcasts that have women sharing their birth stories.

   - VBAC Birth Stories (no longer creating new episodes but their old ones are still available): https://podcasts.apple.com/au/podcast/vbac-birth-stories/id1499980146
   - Australian VBAC Stories: https://podcasts.apple.com/au/podcast/australian-vbac-stories/id1710980590
   - The VBAC Homebirth Stories Podcast: https://themotherhoodcircle.com.au/podcast/
   - The VBAC link Podcast: https://www.thevbaclink.com/podcast/
   - VBAC Babes Podcast: https://linktr.ee/vbacbabes

It's important to remain open minded when reading or listening to their stories. There may be decisions or choices made by women that make you uncomfortable. Recognise that, and then remember their story isn't about you. Finally, remember that EVERY woman deserves respectful maternity care, regardless of their wishes or choices.

Consider the reflective questions below when engaging with the stories.

REFLECTION

When you have read or listened to a VBAC story,

- Where there any parts of the story that made you feel uncomfortable? If so, what where they?

- If you had been part of the woman's story, how do you think she would remember you?

- If the woman made decisions that you feel uncomfortable with, how could have you remained supportive for her?

- Why was her birth option important to her?

Using Positive VBAC Language

In the previous chapter, I discussed using respectful language. Now I want to add using positive VBAC language. Lundgren et al. (2015) explored the views of clinicians in Finland, Sweden, and the Netherlands, countries with high rates of VBAC, on factors influencing VBAC success. Key findings included the importance of a consistent approach to VBAC within the interdisciplinary team, strong collaboration between midwives and obstetricians, and a focus on building trust and alleviating fear among women. Clinicians emphasised the need for a supportive environment that encourages VBAC while prioritising women's safety and respecting their individual choices. One important aspect here is everyone on the team considering VBAC as the first choice. This includes the language used about VBAC. Here is a quote from the study that illustrates this:

The professionals "play" in the same way: they speak the same language, and this talk gradually reaches the woman. This supports successful VBACs, and actually they are mainly very good experiences for the women. (Obstetrician, FI) (Lundgren et al., 2015, p. 5).

Using positive VBAC language isn't disputing that some women will choose to have a repeat caesarean, it's giving information on a safe mode of birth that many women don't know is even an option. It's giving evidence-based care and supporting informed choice. Women are smart enough to take that information and consider the best option for them, if they know about the options in the first place.

Positive VBAC language can start after the first caesarean by informing women that VBAC is an option for the next pregnancy. That may seem premature. However, see it as planting a seed. That seed will grow if it is required and when the time is right the woman will be able to use that information to go and learn more about her birth-after-caesarean choices. If that seed isn't planted, then she may never know that it is an option. Remember the story of Amy at the beginning of Chapter 1?

Clinicians are more likely to encounter women with previous caesareans during their next pregnancies. However, if you work in primary care, you may see women in between pregnancies. That is another great time to use positive VBAC language, if suitable.

During a subsequent pregnancy is the next most important time to use VBAC positive language. This should be available throughout the maternity care system. When a woman speaks to the reception staff to ask for their first appointment, they should be aware of specific birth-after-caesarean clinics or midwifery group practices available. When a woman visits her general practitioner or community doctor, they should be given information on birth-after-caesarean options and providers who support women with previous caesareans.

Since the launch of my first book, I have heard from hundreds of women who found and used the information in the book to have a better birth after caesarean. I remember the story of the woman who went to get her first bloods taken in her pregnancy, and the phlebotomist mentioned VBAC to her and directed her to a birth-after-caesarean clinic at the local hospital. The woman told me she had never heard of VBAC until then. I also remember the story of a woman who was informed about VBAC by the reception staff at the hospital antenatal clinic, and even recommended my book!

During the pregnancy appointments the language should be supportive of VBAC, without the use of coercion. I also think women should be able to make their decision towards the end of their pregnancy, not right at the beginning. Some women know exactly the mode of birth they want from even before the positive pregnancy test, and others need longer to figure out how the pregnancy and baby are going first. Both are valid and women should be able to decide on mode of birth right up to the moment, and even during, labour.

I remember sitting with a couple doing the 36-birth plan appointment in their home. I used a form of art therapy described in my first book, and both the woman and her partner drew their three drawings. As we were finishing up, the woman paused, looked at her drawings, and then ripped them up. She exclaimed that she wanted to change her mind and draw them again. Absolutely! Over another cup of tea and some pizza, she drew a different birth plan from her heart. We discussed it, and made a plan with different options based on what she wanted. It was so cathartic for her and her partner, and her labour and birth resulted in the second birth plan that she drew.

Using positive VBAC language can have a powerful impact. It shows that you have a belief in the importance of vaginal birth, which is in line of what many women believe. It shows that you believe in choice as you will offer and support VBAC, and a caesarean if necessary. I honestly think we can increase our VBAC rates if our interdisciplinary teams of doctors and midwives see VBAC as the first choice, and then support women to be active and upright in labour too. We'll get to active labour in Chapter 8.

"My midwife and I discussed once at the start the 'what if' I was to have an unplanned c section again. What would make it a better experience. Then we never spoke about it again. We were all so determined in making sure I would have my VBAC and having the mindset that it was our only option. I was indeed able to have it!"

CHAPTER 7

How to Support Women to Have a Better Relationship in Their BAC

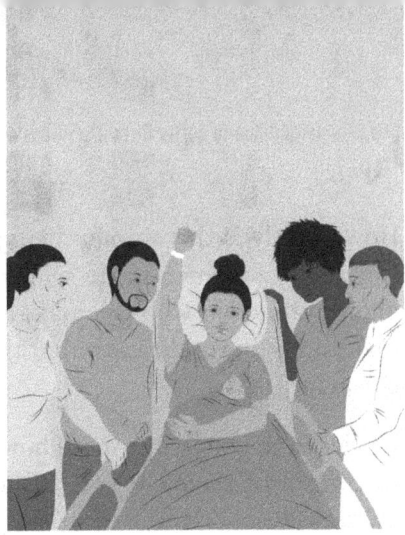

This chapter explores the provider's role in providing relational care based on trust and equity, and how these benefit women planning a better BAC.

In my previous book for women, I started the "relationship factor" with an analogy of choosing their health care provider team like a 100 m sprint Olympic athlete would choose a coach. In short, I suggest that you wouldn't want to choose a coach who didn't believe you would make it to the finish line, and who told you that your body wasn't made for running. I suggest they choose a coach who 100% believes in their ability to beat their personal best and achieve a gold medal, if that is what the athlete wants at the time.

You might be a bit lost now, but just go back to the section on respectful language in Chapter 5 and remember some of the hurtful comment's women received. Look at the comment below and consider how the woman is being made to feel about her body's ability to have a vaginal birth.

> *Resources wasted on me, time waster, accept my body won't birth, I'm also sick to death of terminology like unfavourable cervix, failure to progress, overactive uterus like I'm deformed and broken. I just don't like being prodded and pricked like a science experiment! I don't want to birth in that atmosphere and I'm unique. Not average!* (PP370, Public hospital care). (Keedle et al., 2022, p. 8).

How exactly is this woman being supported by her health care team? I encourage women to be selective about their health care team and choose clinicians who will make a great support team. I suggest that you focus on being a clinician that the woman won't regret bringing onto their team.

Earlier in the book, I covered how you can support women to feel more in control of their choices, wishes, and outcomes, and how you can increase your confidence in supporting women. This includes knowing the evidence, not using coercion, and taking time to understand women's stories and wishes for their births.

"I think the key there is in the question. How can they support you to have the best birth after caesarean that YOU want? It shouldn't be about their agenda, and if they don't feel confident or capable to support you the way you want to be supported, they should be swallowing their pride to refer you to someone who will. Women should be provided with quality evidence-based information to assist them in decision making, free of coercion or professional bias, and supported in their decision that they then make. It's their right to do so. Be the coach that believes in them and helps them over the finish line."

Models of Care

Clinicians should be aware of the different models of maternity care available, including continuity of care (CoC) and standard fragmented care. Midwifery CoC is a model where the same midwife provides care throughout pregnancy, labour and birth, and for up to 6 weeks postpartum. There are numerous studies and systematic reviews that show this model has many benefits for women, including a lower likelihood of episiotomies, caesarean and instrumental births, and a higher chance of a spontaneous vaginal birth, as well as women having a more positive experience (Sandall et al., 2024).

Studies have also shown that midwifery CoC can be beneficial for women planning a VBAC. A study from China found that women who had midwifery CoC had shorter labours, less postpartum haemorrhage, and higher VBAC rates compared to women who received standard care (88% compared to 68% in the standard care group) (Zhang & Liu, 2016).

The quality of CoC is important. An Australian study compared midwifery CoC to standard care, and found that women in both models reported seeing multiple midwives during their pregnancy and labour (Homer et al., 2021). This lack of continuity may have contributed to no significant difference in VBAC rates between the two groups. A separate small study from Australia found women who had midwifery CoC were 2.48 times more likely to have a VBAC compared to no continuity of care (Facchetti et al., 2024). The same study found private obstetrician CoC models decreased the likelihood of VBAC success compared to no continuity of care (RR 0.69) (Facchetti et al., 2024).

In my PhD paper comparing the experiences of women planning a VBAC in midwifery CoC, private obstetric CoC, and standard fragmented care we found that:

> Women who had CoC with a midwife were more likely to feel in control of their decision making, and feel their health care provider positively supported their decision to have a VBAC. Women who had CoC with a midwife were more likely to have been active in labour, experience water immersion, and have an upright birthing position. Women who received fragmented care experienced lower autonomy and lower respect compared to CoC (Keedle et al., 2020a, p. 1).

One variable we explored was the length of time for antenatal appointments under the different models of care, with the understanding that it takes time to develop relationships with women that are based on trust, empathy, and respect (Keedle et al., 2020a). Our findings demonstrated that women in midwifery CoC had, on average, longer appointments with women (30 to 60 mins) compared to private obstetric CoC and standard care (10 to 15 mins). This was also demonstrated in a Japanese study that found longer appointments and higher satisfaction scores in midwife-led care compared to doctor-led care (Iida et al., 2014). There is much more to the professional relationship between women and clinicians than the amount of time spent in appointments, but it certainly has an impact. The increased time allows for more time to develop a relationship and provide emotional support.

In our national maternity experiences study, we asked women what they would do differently in a subsequent study. We focused on models of care. In that category, 62% of comments were women stated that they would choose a midwifery continuity of care model, 16% of women stated private obstetric care, and 3% stated using the public fragmented system (Keedle et al., 2023). It's fair to say that midwifery CoC not only has better maternal outcomes, but that women want to have access to that model of care.

This may sound like I have a bias for midwifery CoC, and in a way, I do. I have worked in midwifery CoC models in both public settings and as a private midwife. I have seen these benefits for myself. However, I am a researcher and academic and I'm passionate about presenting evidence-based information to clinicians and women. It is the first Standard of Practice for Midwives in Australia: Promotes health and wellbeing through evidence-based midwifery practice (NMBA, 2018).

If you are a midwife working in CoC, thank you for committing to work in an evidence-based model of care that epitomises woman-centred care. If you are a student midwife, please consider working in that model when you qualify. If you are a midwife not working in that model, then maybe consider moving into that model. It's very different from shift work, but it provides many advantages. Australia is experiencing a growth in midwifery models of care, and it's very exciting to see our Federal and State Parliaments supporting midwifery. There is a long way to go, but we are certainly doing better than before in expanding midwifery models of care.

However, if you are a doctor or other clinician, you are not being excluded from maternity care by the promotion of midwifery CoC. It is imperative that women have access to a collaborative and integrated team. One professional cannot provide everything a woman may need. Midwives need to have seamless referral pathways with obstetricians, physiotherapists, mental health professionals, and community health, to name a few. As a clinician, your support of evidence- based models of care is vital to the success of them. The maternity care team is stronger together with respectful communication, and recognition of our scope of practice and skills.

One of our BESt papers explored the strengths and limitations of models of care from women's perspectives. Private obstetric care was stronger when they worked in collaboration within a multidisciplinary team, which included access to midwifery care. Another strength of private obstetric care was knowledge around high-risk pregnancies (Pelak et al., 2023).

This same paper found a limitation to midwifery CoC was when there wasn't the level of support or connection that they were hoping to from their midwife (Pelak et al., 2023). It is important that clinicians have strategies in place when the relationship isn't beneficial for the woman or themselves. A New Zealand study found this was a complex area and was uncertain about how to manage these relationships. The midwives gave strategies, such as having difficult conversations with the aim for resolution or referring their clients onto another clinician (James, 2020).

If you provide continuity of care, what strategies do you have in place if the professional relationship between yourself and a woman is not beneficial? I suggest you reflect on this question. I definitely think research should be done on this challenging aspect of CoC.

Providing Trustworthy Care

In Chapter 5, I presented the values of trauma-informed care. Trustworthiness was one of the values. Women who trust their clinicians are more likely to have a better relationship with their clinician in their next birth after caesarean. The Integrated Trauma-Informed Care Framework developed by NSW Health describes the value of trustworthiness as:

> *Service providers and clinicians are transparent, and seek to build and maintain trust among clients, staff, and other services. Being trustworthy involves being reliable, accountable, respecting boundaries, and not sharing information that is not yours to share. It takes time and effort to build trust particularly where trust has been broken* (NSW Health, 2023, p. 20).

This definition is a helpful yardstick to measure the care you provide. Are you transparent about the information you provide and the suggestions you give? Are you reliable? Many women find clinicians practice bait and switch. This is when the clinician appears supportive of the woman's birth choice, usually a VBAC (the bait), and then show a change in this support, such as booking a repeat caesarean without adequate explanation or reason (the switch) (Reyes Foster, 2023). This shows a lack of transparency and reliability, which leads to mistrust between the woman and the clinician.

"Expect that VBAC women don't trust you. You need to work hard to gain their trust because they were likely once bitten and twice shy.

Stop commenting on my fricken' pelvis and its hypothetical size or that it's "un-tested." Stop inflating the risks because you're scared. I had to educate myself, I expect you do so too. What makes you feel more comfortable doesn't mean it makes me feel more comfortable."

Fear-Based Care

It is also important to discuss the impact of fear-based care. Fear can originate from a previous personal or professional experience, or from the wider impact of peer expectations. It can also eventuate from fearing the impact of a poor outcome. This can lead to practising in a defensive manner to maintain control and pre-empt legal issues (Smith-Oka, 2022).

A qualitative study of 12 obstetric doctors in Mexico found:

> ... they saw pregnant bodies as inherently risky, and birth as having to be tightly controlled for fear of an unexpected emergency. These perceptions appeared to be based on two primary factors—that the hospital attended to a high proportion of high-risk births, and the circulation among the trainees of 'war stories' describing bad experiences that their colleagues had had. According to Pablo, a fourth-year resident, 'All patients have risk from the moment they become pregnant'" (Smith-Oka, 2022, p. 3).

Fear can be paralysing and cloud your judgement and actions. When I was writing this chapter, the epic BBC *Call the Midwife* series 14, set in 1970, was released. In episode 1, a pregnant woman called Winnie is told she must have a repeat caesarean following her previous caesarean with a visible vertical caesarean abdominal scar. Winnie is in the hospital and the team of doctors and students are informing her of this decision.

Later in the episode, Winnie sees the midwife Nurse Crane, and it seems that she is traumatised from her previous caesarean experience, but she is also terrified of having a uterine rupture. Nurse Crane reinforces the need for her to have a repeat caesarean. In a later scene, Nurse Crane discloses to Nurse Clifford that she witnessed a woman die following a uterine rupture at home and she concludes, "The fact of the matter is, if there is any risk at all of uterine rupture, the knife is the only way ahead."

In pure dramatic fashion, Winnie goes into labour at home during a protest in her area that blocks the road. The Nonnatus House midwives, Nurse Crane and Nurse Clifford, walk through the protest to support Winnie. In the home of Winnie, she is close to birthing her baby and Nurse Clifford supports her. Nurse Crane freezes. I think it's a powerful scene as this is uncharacteristic of Nurse Crane, a very experienced nurse midwife. Nurse Clifford prompts Nurse Crane to call for the flying squad (ambulance), and Winnie goes ahead and births her baby vaginally at home.

It seems that for Nurse Crane she needed support from a colleague and the experience of seeing that not all previous caesareans result in a uterine rupture, even one with a vertical scar. The storyline also showed that you can have those fears, but you don't have to share them with the woman, as Nurse Crane discusses in her disclosure scene. I wonder if Nurse Crane's actions would have been different if there had been access to talking therapies and debriefing more than 40 years ago. Mind you, has the culture really changed regarding getting support and help?

I confess that I have been a fan of the *Call the Midwife* series since it started in 2012. Nurse Crane reminds me so much of my Granny who was a midwife in the UK during that time. She even did her midwife training in that area of East London before moving back to Buckinghamshire where she worked as a District Midwife for many years.

The journey from fear to trust is a challenging one, and there is little research that I could find on this. Personally, I have found increasing knowledge to be beneficial, especially when you have experienced a rare obstetric event, such as a uterine rupture or an amniotic fluid embolism. Getting therapeutic support, such as counselling or psychotherapy, may also be required. As a clinician, you need to be providing evidence-based, not fear-based care as this will impact your support for women negatively.

> "I can appreciate that OBs and midwives have no doubt seen and dealt with some horrible situations. I am sure those memories haunt them. But please don't bring that into my birth. Don't project your fears onto me. Don't tell me that you've seen worst-case scenarios, and that it happens more than I think. Don't dismiss current and up-to-date research because of these experiences. And please don't disassociate from me and my birth for fear of the choices I've made."

> ### REFLECTION
>
> Supporting women by having a better relationship.
>
> - Reflecting on the trustworthiness section of this chapter, do you feel that your practice encourages women's trust? Are there areas you could improve on? What areas are your strengths? Why is that?
>
> Reflecting on the fear-based care section of this chapter, do you feel you practice fear-based care with women? How does that make you feel? How will you approach that?

Doulas

Doula support during labour and birth provides numerous evidence-based benefits for women and their families. Doulas provide continuous emotional and physical support to women and their partners during labour and birth. Although not registered health care professionals, doulas undergo specialised training and certification to provide evidence-based support.

Studies have shown that doula support can lead to reduced caesarean rates, decreased use of epidurals and other pain medications, shorter labour durations, and reduced length of hospital stay (Adams & Curtin-Bowen, 2021; Bohren et al., 2017; Kozhimannil & Hardeman, 2016). Doula support has also been linked to increased confidence in birthing and parenting abilities, development of trusting relationships with the doula and support team, improved decision-making and informed choices, and a positive impact on emotional well-being (Akhavan & Edge, 2012; Byrskog et al., 2020; Darwin et al., 2017; Kozhimannil et al., 2016; McGarry et al., 2016; McLeish & Redshaw, 2019; Thomas et al., 2017)

These benefits extend to diverse populations, including migrant women (Akhavan & Edge, 2012; Oommen et al., 2024), women with low socioeconomic status (Darwin et al., 2017), women of colour

(Hardeman & Kozhimannil, 2016; Mottl-Santiago et al., 2023), women with intellectual disabilities (McGarry et al., 2016), and women in prison (Shlafer et al., 2021).

A scoping review of 25 studies examined the utilisation of doula-support services among birthing people of colour in the United States (Kang et al., 2024). As discussed in Chapter 5, women of colour experience higher rates of adverse birth outcomes compared to white women. This review found that despite the potential benefits, doula support services are underutilised by this population due to limited awareness and access. The benefits of doula support included giving confidence to women of colour to have more agency in the maternity system, providing information and education on the perinatal period, and through advocating for women. Two of the studies found a decrease in preterm birth rates, and two studies found a decrease in caesarean births and increased breast-feeding initiation (Kang et al., 2024).

A study from Norway evaluated the impact of a Multicultural Doula (MCD) program on obstetric and neonatal outcomes for newly arrived migrant women (Oommen et al., 2024). Compared to women without MCD support, those who received it demonstrated a 41% lower likelihood of emergency caesarean sections, and a 75% lower risk of significant blood loss during vaginal birth. Additionally, MCD support was associated with increased use of non-pharmacological and pharmacological pain relief during labour and higher rates of exclusive breastfeeding at discharge. These findings suggest that MCD programs may significantly improve maternal outcomes for migrant women (Oommen et al., 2024).

I do think clinicians should acknowledge the value of doula support, inform women about their benefits, facilitate collaboration between doulas and the clinical team, and address access barriers to doula support.

"Encourage your clients to book a doula! Build a network of doulas you regularly work with and refer patients to them. They are worth their weight in gold!!

Also support them in choosing to advocate for their own wishes when they're research backed but against hospital policy. My amazing midwife made it so easy for me, having all the forms I needed to sign ready at my request, to not have cervical checks, cannula or CTG, and then kept the doctors out of the room so I could have an uninterrupted, incredible water birth. I'm so grateful!"

CHAPTER 8

How to Support Women to be Active in Labour When Planning a VBAC

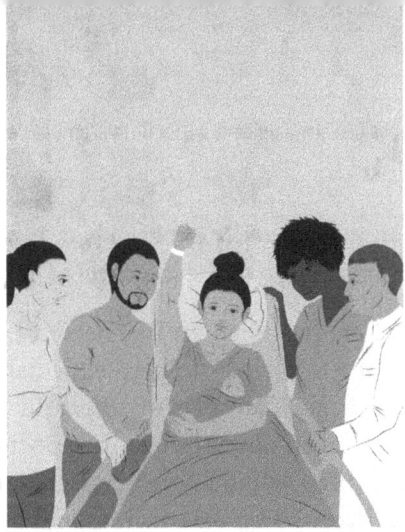

Remember the birth plans reflection in Chapter 5? In this reflection, I prompted you to explore what your birth preferences were. The following questions were included:

> How do you imagine your ideal labour and birth? If you were to draw this, what would be there? What environment are you birthing in? Who is there? What are you using in labour to help with the challenging waves of contractions? What's your birthing position?

In that reflection, I suggested that you think about these to help you become aware of the biases so that you can support a woman who envisions something different.

As a clinical midwife, I used the ideal-birth-scenario art practice with women and their partners during pregnancy. I also used the practice in childbirth education classes offered through a hospital. These childbirth education classes helped me understand the vast gap between what women were imagining and what they may actually experience during labour and birth. The women mostly drew themselves upright and mobilising, or in birthing pools. There was darkness, privacy, music, and only a few people that they chose to be in the room. Based on the increasing rates of intervention, and the impact of the clinicians following prescriptive policies and guidelines, I can only imagine what these women actually experienced. Is their reaction due to their high expectations or due to the low level of care and support they received?

There has been an increase in the discourse around the "problem" of women having too high expectations in the maternity academic space and media, especially here in Australia following the NSW Birth Trauma inquiry. Indeed, one doctor gave evidence at one of the hearings blaming women's high expectations for their traumatic births. The idea is that women have unreasonably high expectations and when interventions are used that result in them having unexpected birth outcomes, and feeling traumatised about them, then it is their fault. I suggest there is another term for this: victim blaming.

I know that women's high expectations are not causing birth trauma because I have seen the powerful and healing side of birth. I have seen women use their surroundings, support people, and their bodies to make an oxytocin-rich environment that gives them the support they need. I have seen women have the birth that they drew their ideal birth and their expectations were matched, and often exceeded.

Clinicians play a key role during intrapartum care. They are often the gatekeepers that determine whether a woman experiences a positive or negative labour and birth. The World Health Organization defines a positive childbirth experience as:

> ... one that fulfils or exceeds a woman's prior personal and socio-cultural beliefs and expectations, including giving birth to a healthy baby in a clinically and psychologically safe environment with continuity of practical and emotional support from a birth companion(s) and kind, technically competent clinical staff. It is based on the premise that most women want a physiological labour and birth, and to have a sense of personal achievement and control through involvement in decision-making, even when medical interventions are needed or wanted (WHO, 2018, p. 1).

To bring it back, if women want to plan a VBAC, they need to be supported during labour and birth. We know there is a small risk of uterine rupture. However, we need to recognise that women need clinicians who are willing to support them to increase their chance of having vaginal births. Many of these women know the factors associated with having a vaginal birth. After reading Chapter 6, you will have directed them to evidence-based resources to increase their knowledge. This may include attending classes that focus on hypnobirthing, yoga, or acupressure. In my PhD VBAC survey, we found that 30% of women accessed alternative therapy education classes (Keedle et al., 2020a).

Being upright and active in labour and birth has a positive impact on the experience of labour and vaginal birth. Most birth positions involve restricted movement, with women lying on their backs during labour. However, research strongly supports the benefits of active labour, including walking, upright positions, and movement.

A Cochrane Review found that upright positions in the first stage of labour can reduce labour duration, the risk of caesarean section, and the need for epidural anaesthesia (Lawrence et al., 2013). Conversely, remaining recumbent increases the likelihood of interventions, such as assisted births and synthetic oxytocin.

My PhD VBAC study found that women who were active during labour, regardless of the birth outcome, felt more empowered and resolved (Keedle et al., 2020a). This aligns with findings that active labour, including position changes, breathing techniques, and using the shower, contributes to a more positive birth experience (Kibuka et al., 2021).

As clinicians, we have an immense impact on how this environment is used to facilitate or inhibit women's labour and birth experience. Let's explore birth environment.

Birth Environment

Research has explored the impact of the birth environment on maternal and infant well-being. Factors, such as oxytocin levels, stress, and the overall quality of care significantly influence birth outcomes (Walter et al., 2021). Studies have shown that supportive environments that minimise stress, prioritise women's autonomy, and foster positive relationships can lead to improved outcomes, such as increased rates of vaginal birth and enhanced maternal-infant bonding (Migliorini et al., 2023).

A multicentre randomised-controlled trial from Germany investigated the impact of a specially designed hospital birthing room on vaginal birth rates (Ayerle et al., 2023). The intervention room was designed to encourage mobility, self-determination, and upright maternal positions by removing the bed and providing alternative equipment.

While there was a slight increase in vaginal birth rates in the intervention group, the difference was not statistically significant. Secondary outcomes (episiotomy, perineal tears, epidural use, neonatal outcomes), nor serious adverse events differed between groups (Ayerle et al., 2023). However, the study found a strong association between upright maternal positions and maternal self-determination, regardless of room assignment. The researchers concluded that the increased vaginal birth rates in both groups were likely due to high motivation among women and staff rather than the specific features of the intervention room.

An ethnographic study from Sweden explored the influence of the birth environment on nulliparous women giving birth in two differently designed hospital rooms (Goldkuhl et al., 2022). Findings revealed that while physical space plays a role, the dominant factor was the "Birth Manual"—an implicit set of institutional rules and expectations that guided labour management. This resulted in two contrasting experiences: an "Institutional Room," where women felt passive and subject to medical interventions, and a more "Personal room," where agency was facilitated.

The study highlights that even with variations in room design, the pervasive influence of institutional authority can undermine women's autonomy and control over their birth experience. The researchers emphasise the critical role of a supportive birth philosophy in creating safe and empowering environments that prioritise women's needs and agency (Goldkuhl et al., 2022).

A study from Malta explored the lived experiences of women and their male partners during childbirth at a public hospital (Mizzi & Pace Parascandalo, 2022). Using an interpretive phenomenological approach, the researchers investigated how the physical, psychosocial, spiritual, and cultural aspects of the birth environment influenced parental experiences.

The study findings revealed a "home-hospital gap," where the clinical setting, despite efforts to create a home-like atmosphere, felt foreign and unsettling to both parents. The quality of midwifery care emerged as a crucial factor, overshadowing the impact of the physical environment.

It also found that women prioritised movement during labour and their male partners reported increased involvement when women were mobile. The study highlights the importance of creating an environment that facilitates movement and minimises constraints on parental agency (Mizzi & Pace Parascandalo, 2022).

Key considerations for creating optimal birth environments include minimising stress, empowering women, fostering positive relationships, and supporting midwives (Ayerle et al., 2023; Goldkuhl et al., 2022; Murray-Davis et al., 2023).

In summary, the research underscores the multifaceted nature of the birth environment and its impact on maternal and infant well-being. While physical aspects like room design and available resources play a role, the human element, including the quality of midwifery care, the extent of women's autonomy, and the overall hospital culture, have a larger impact.

Further research is needed to fully understand the complex interplay between these factors and to develop evidence-based interventions that optimise the birth experience for all women.

Methods to Remain Active in Labour

There are a variety of methods to remain active and encourage mobility during labour. Many women use an exercise ball during pregnancy and research has explored the use of the exercise ball during labour. Systematic reviews on the use of birthing balls found their use significantly reduced maternal pain during labour although didn't impact mode of birth (Grenvik et al., 2022). A systematic review that included the use of the peanut ball and birthing balls found there use contributed to a reduced duration of the first stage of labour, and an increase in vaginal births with no difference in complications (Grenvik et al., 2023). Both reviews suggest that using birthing balls and peanut balls during labour can have positive effects.

A randomised-controlled trial from Turkey evaluated the impact of hypnobirthing training on fear of childbirth, pain, and birth outcomes in 80 nulliparous women (Buran & Aksu, 2022). Women in the hypno-birthing group participated in weekly group sessions, resulting in significantly lower fear of childbirth scores, reduced pain perception throughout labour, fewer interventions, shorter delivery times, higher rates of vaginal birth, and greater birth satisfaction compared to the control group. These findings suggest that hypnobirthing can be a valu-able non-pharmacological pain management strategy.

Guidelines recommend women planning a VBAC to use continuous foetal monitoring (ACOG, 2019). However, women can find the use of the CTG as restrictive during labour. Fox et al. (2024) explored Australian women's and birthing people's experiences with foetal monitoring during labour through a national survey. A qualitative analysis of the open text responses revealed two key themes: "Tending to the machine" and "Impressions of the machine." "Tending to the machine" highlighted instances where clinicians prioritised monitoring equipment over the individual's needs and preferences, often overlooking the impact of restrictions on freedom of movement. "Impressions of the machine" emphasised how the physical constraints of monitoring devices can negatively impact labour progress and the overall birth experience.

The study highlighted the need for clinicians to provide more compre-hensive information about foetal monitoring options, including their potential impact on labour and the individual's experience (Fox et al., 2024). Prioritising the individual's needs and minimising the constraints imposed by monitoring technologies are crucial for providing high-quality, woman-centred intrapartum care.

The following section has been written by Dr. Kirsten Small regarding the use of the CTG for women planning a VBAC. Thank you, Kirsten, for supplying this important information.

VBAC and the CTG for Maternity Professionals

Dr Kirsten Small is an obstetrically trained researcher and educator, with a PhD in foetal monitoring. Her blog, www.birthsmalltalk.com, provides a large collection of useful and free resources about the evidence for different approaches to foetal heart rate monitoring in labour.

All foetal monitoring guidelines produced by major professional organisations (such as NICE, ACOG, and RANZCOG) advise the use of CTG monitoring during labour for women with a history of one or more caesarean sections. What evidence supports this recommendation?

Only one randomised-controlled trial has recruited women with a history of one prior caesarean section to help answer this question (Madaan & Trivedi, 2006). The trial was conducted in India in 2006. Women were randomly assigned to either intermittent auscultation or continuous CTG monitoring, with no information provided about whether external or internal monitoring, or telemetry were used. No babies died during the trial, and there were no significant differences in Apgar scores of less than 7 at one and 5 minutes of age, rates of admission to neonatal intensive care, or "birth asphyxia" (how this was diagnosed was not defined). This is not altogether surprising as the trial had only 50 women in each arm—far too small to detect a meaningful difference if one existed. There was also (again, unsurprising due to the small number of women) no statistically significant difference in the mode of birth, though the rate of repeat caesarean section was 22% in the intermittent auscultation group, and 34% in the CTG-monitoring group. The size of this rise is consistent with the increase in caesarean section seen in other randomised- controlled trials about CTG use.

There is, therefore, no good quality evidence to be confident about whether CTG use, rather than intermittent auscultation, makes anything better, or worse, for women who have previously had one caesarean section or their babies. There is no direct evidence at all to guide foetal monitoring decisions for women who have had more than one caesarean section. No legitimate argument can be made that women considered to be at high-risk benefit from CTG use in labour, as evidence from randomised-controlled trials in high-risk populations shows no better outcomes (Alfirevic et al., 2017). This is reinforced by evidence generated using other research approaches (Small et al., 2020).

It is sometimes argued that CTG monitoring is superior to intermittent auscultation as it can predict when uterine rupture is about to happen or permit earlier detection of uterine rupture once it has occurred. There is some, but not much, research comparing foetal heart rate patterns for women over the hours prior to a diagnosis of uterine rupture where a control group of women who have had a prior caesarean section was used.

Andersen et al. (2016) looked at this in a Danish population, with the only significant difference in heart rate patterns being the presence of at least 10 severe variable decelerations in a 30-minute period. Similar research in France (Desseauve et al., 2016) found foetal bradycardia to be the most common abnormal pattern seen, with heart-rate traces classified as abnormal occurring for 81% of women with uterine rupture and 25% of those without rupture. There is, therefore, no heart-rate pattern that clearly distinguishes the impending or already present situation of uterine rupture from the range of causes for abnormal heart-rate patterns in labours that are not complicated by rupture.

While both these studies used CTG recordings, this does not mean that the same patterns would have remained undetected if intermittent auscultation were in use. Foetal bradycardia and repeated severe decelerations are likely to be readily apparent on intermittent auscultation. The absence of difference in perinatal outcomes in research comparing CTG use with intermittent auscultation in women without prior caesarean section suggests that clinically significant heart rate abnormalities are rarely overlooked with intermittent auscultation (Alfirevic et al., 2017; Heelan Fancher et al., 2019).

The presence of a risk factor, such as prior caesarean section, does not remove the need to obtain informed consent prior to the use of any form of foetal heart rate monitoring. The RANZCOG Foetal Surveillance guideline specifically recommends that women be given information about foetal-monitoring options, in addition to advising that women be offered CTG monitoring for VBAC (RANZCOG, 2019c). Local hospital policy that mandates the "required" use of CTG monitoring for women during VBAC undermines human rights principles and should be challenged (Small et al., 2023). It is vital that women are given factual evidence—scaremongering approaches, such as implying that perinatal mortality rates are higher when intermittent auscultation is in use, are unethical.

When women do choose to use CTG monitoring for their VBAC, it can be challenging to support freedom of movement. Telemetry appears to facilitate more mobility during labour (Watson et al., 2022). Some midwives find the combination of a foetal spiral electrode and waterproof telemetry facilitates continuous CTG monitoring during water immersion. New non-invasive foetal ECG monitoring is both beltless and wireless, using stick on patches. Women report greater freedom of movement (Coddington et al., 2023) and midwives describe less time spent adjusting sensors (D. Fox et al., 2021). For each of these options, no research has examined whether the use of these alternatives to standard "wired" CTG monitoring has any impact on perinatal outcomes or the mode of birth.

There is a new device for foetal monitoring that is being researched. Deborah Fox et al. (2021) investigated the feasibility of using a new wireless and beltless foetal monitoring device (NIFECG) in a clinical setting for the entire duration of labour. The device utilises foetal and maternal electrocardiography, and uterine electromyography. Findings demonstrated that women appreciated the comfort and freedom of movement afforded by NIFECG. Midwives reported that when the signal was stable, the device allowed them to focus more on women's emotional and physical needs. While clinicians recognised the benefits for women, concerns were raised regarding the reliability of the foetal heart rate signal, particularly during signal loss (Fox et al., 2021).

This study provides valuable insights into the feasibility and potential of NIFECG as an alternative to traditional cardiotocography (CTG) for foetal monitoring. Further research and technological advancements to address signal reliability are crucial to determine the long-term clinical utility of this promising technology. There is also the limitation of the device not being waterproof, and therefore being unable to use when the women wish to use water immersion.

Water Immersion and Waterbirth

There is growing research that highlights the benefits of water immersion during labour and birth, including improved freedom of movement, enhanced pain relief, increased relaxation, and potential for shorter labours (Carlsson & Ulfsdottir, 2020; Cooper & Warland, 2019; Hodgson et al., 2020). Studies have shown that women who use water immersion often experience a greater sense of control and empowerment (Clews et al., 2019; Fair et al., 2020).

Recently Australian researcher Beth Townsend completed her PhD by studying women's experiences of water immersion and planning a VBAC. This grounded-theory study explored women's experiences of negotiating water immersion during labour for VBAC (Townsend et al., 2023). Findings revealed that "taking the reins" was the core category, emphasising women's active role in advocating for their birth preferences. Driven by a desire for a "natural and normal" birth, women actively sought information and navigated the health care system to access water immersion. Key factors influencing their success included having strong support from other women and continuity of midwifery care. However, navigating institutional "Rules for birth" often presented significant challenges. This study highlights the importance of acknowledging women's agency, supporting their informed decision-making, and creating a more collaborative and woman-centred approach to VBAC care (Townsend et al., 2023).

Water immersion can be a valuable option for women planning a VBAC, particularly with the availability of wireless CTG monitoring. Importantly, research suggests that water birth poses no increased risk of harm to the baby compared to land birth. While home births often involve inflatable pools, many hospitals and birth centres offer purpose-built deep baths.

It is crucial to explore why many clinicians create barriers for women accessing waterbirth. An Australian study explored midwives' experiences with water immersion for labour and birth, focusing on how policies and guidelines influence their practice (Cooper et al., 2021). Findings revealed a complex interplay of factors, including systemic constraints, external pressures from other health care professionals, and the limitations of existing policies, that can significantly impact midwives' ability to offer and women's access to water immersion. These factors often restrict midwifery autonomy and can inadvertently limit woman-centred care. The study emphasises the need to critically examine existing policies and guidelines to ensure they truly support woman-centred care and empower midwives to fully utilise their expertise and clinical judgment (Cooper et al., 2021). By addressing these challenges, we can work towards creating a more supportive and empowering environment for both midwives and women during labour and birth.

Birthing Positions

There are psychological and physiological benefits to upright birthing positions that allow the sacrum to be flexible compared to reclining positions that restrict the sacrum. However, most women in hospital birth on their back or in a semi-sitting position (Satone & Tayade, 2023; Scholten et al., 2024). Although many women during the pregnancy wish to birth in an upright position (Kjeldsen et al., 2022). A study of 447 women from Denmark found 71% of pregnant women wished to birth in a sacrum flexible position (squat, all fours, standing, birthstool, waterbirth). However, 86% of these women birthed in a non-flexible sacrum position (supine or lying on side) (Kjeldsen et al., 2022). The researchers surmised that the culture of the birth environment and the experience and attitude of the clinicians had an influential impact on the birth position.

A study from Germany found 78% of women birthed in the supine position, and many stated that women did not choose this position. The regression model found women who birthed in a supine position had less satisfaction with their birth experiences (Scholten et al., 2024).

A qualitative study from Saudi Arabia explored clinicians' perspectives around using upright birth positions. The study found clinicians preferred to use the lithotomy positions based on their own comfort and convenience, and this took precedence over the woman's preference for an upright birthing position (Murshed Alsehimi & Shaban, 2021).

This is quite negative to read, but certainly highlights the challenge women have, to birth in a position that they choose. It also highlights the influential role the clinician has during labour and birth.

You can change this. Practice evidence-based care by supporting women to birth in different positions. If you are not confident in this, then ask for support and mentoring from those that are.

I remember supporting a woman who wanted to birth standing up and leaning on a bed. She was doing amazingly, and the baby was descending well. Her private obstetrician came in and squatted down next to me. He whispered to me that he hadn't supported a standing birth. I told him to take my lead, and he can learn. It was wonderful that he was able to collaborate with me and not force the woman to change her birthing position and the standing birth was a great experience for the woman and her support team. The upsetting part was that this was his last year working as an obstetrician before he retired. All those years, and this was his first standing birth.

Challenge yourself. Learn from those that are confident and become a clinician that can support women to be active in labour.

Have a look at the following images on how you can support women to be upright and active in labour for ideas.

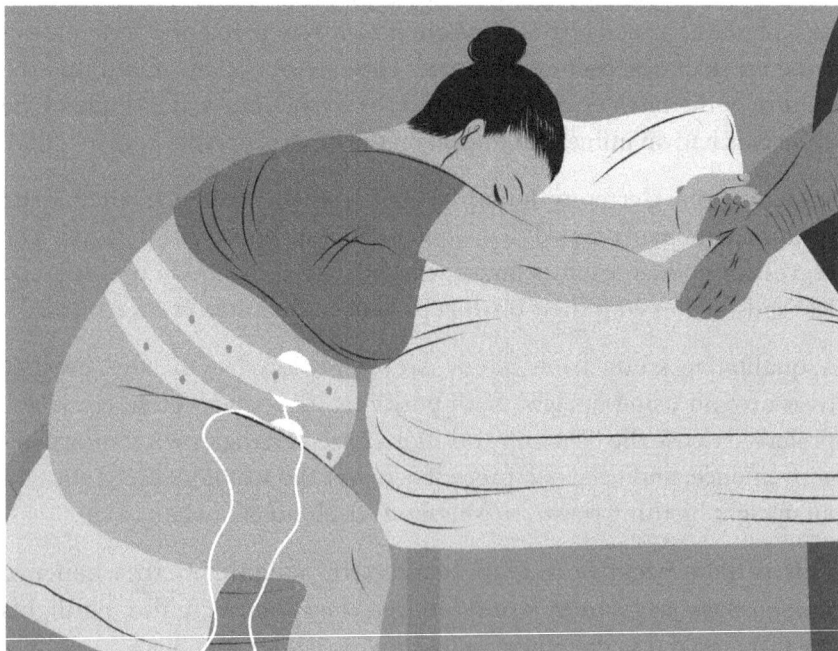

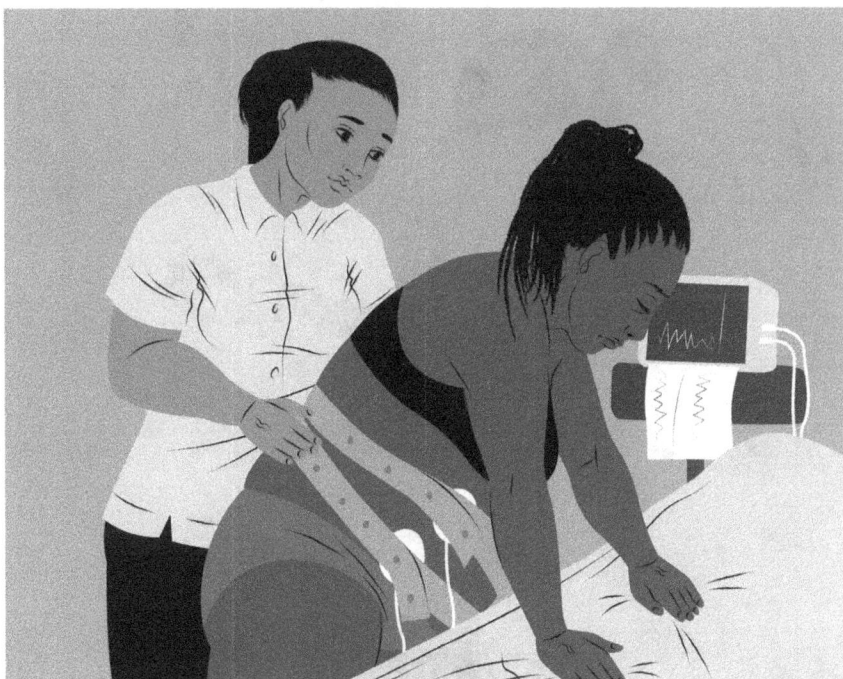

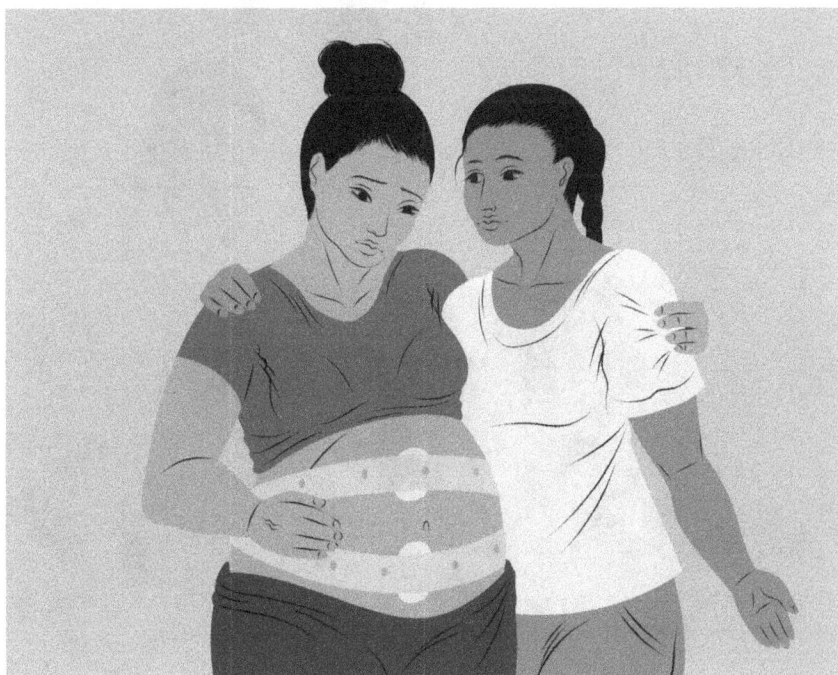

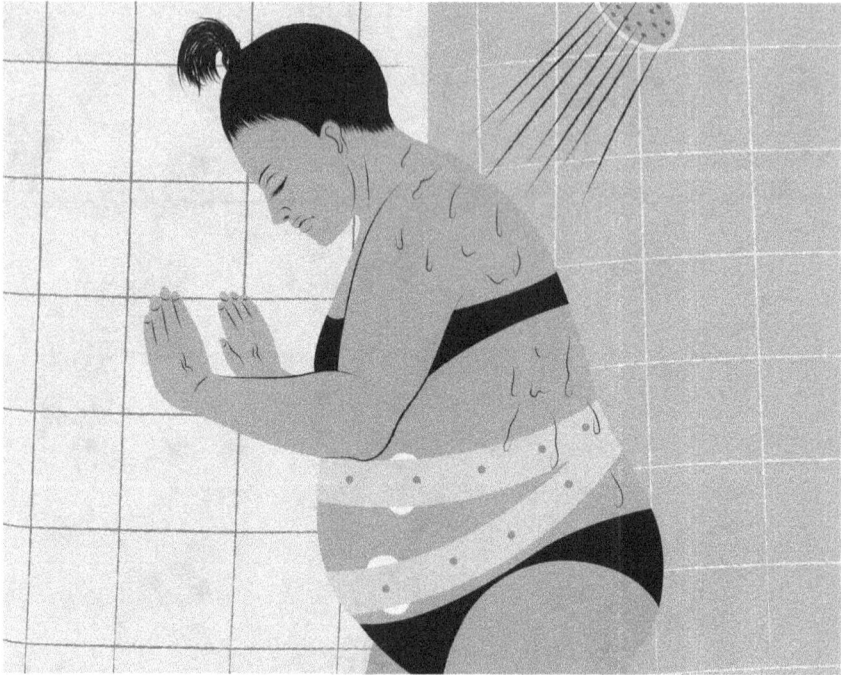

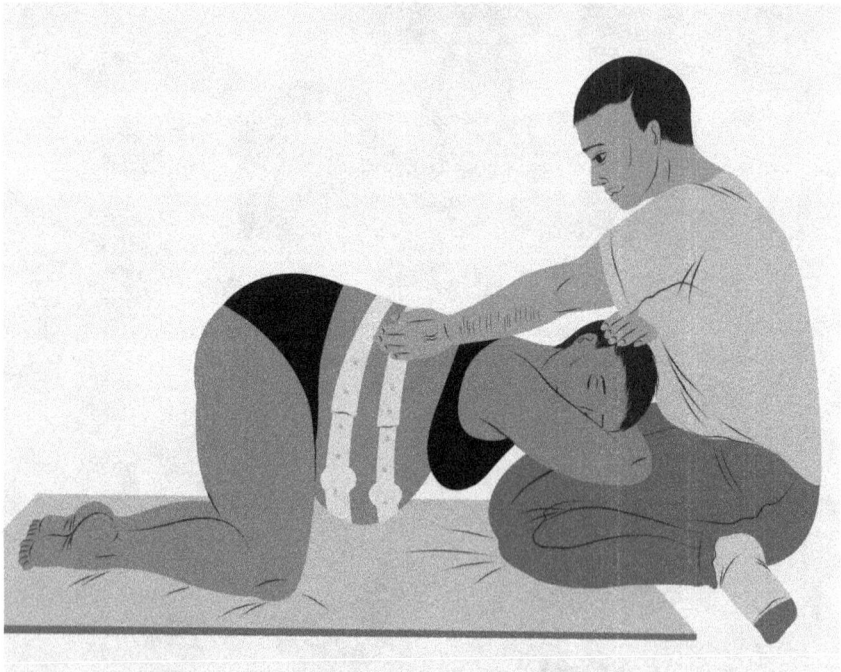

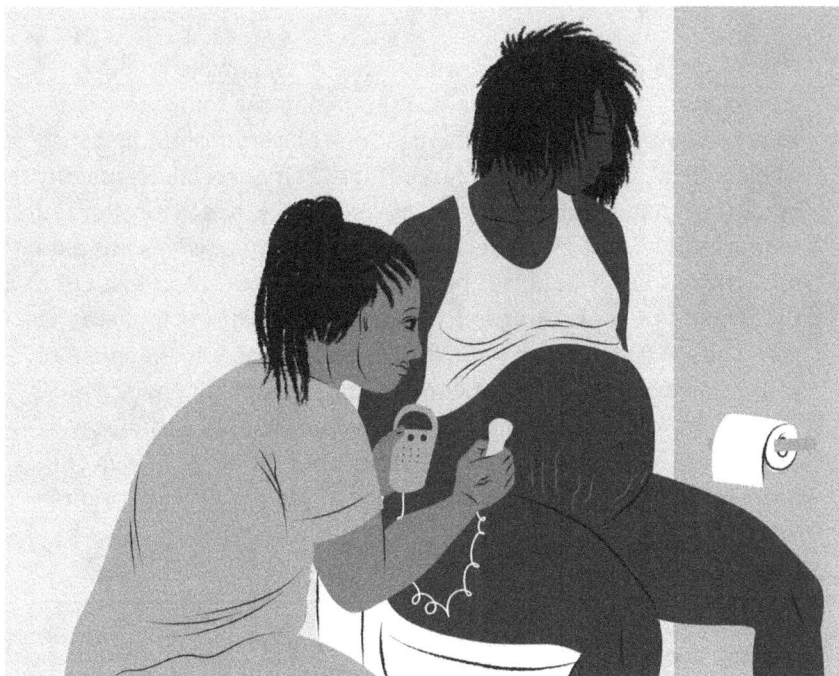

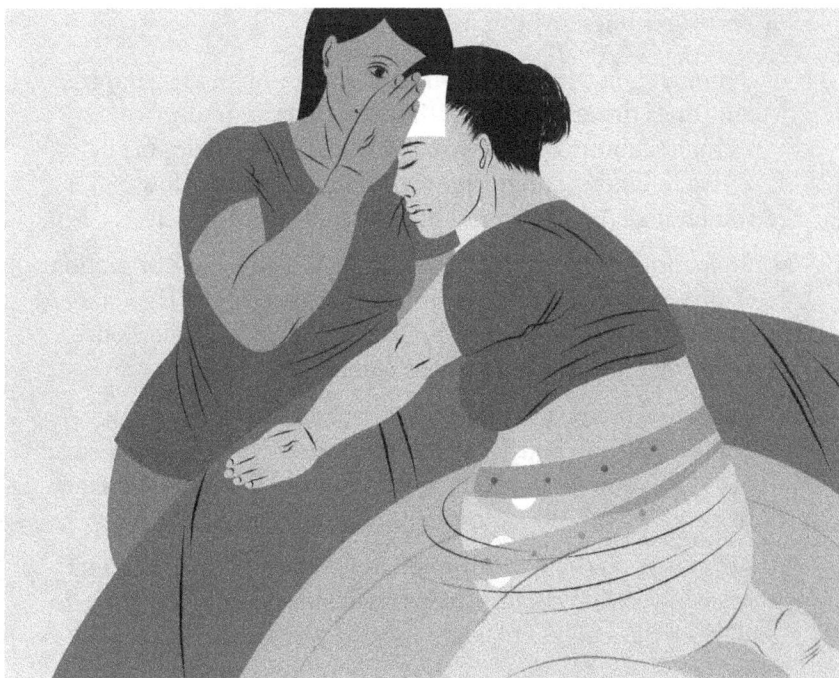

"Start from a position of yes, a baseline of "let's make this happen". Then assess as you go, taking the individual, their specific circumstances for THIS pregnancy, and their whole self as the priority focus, rather than generalised, mostly outdated, policy/guidelines, which is usually based on limited research findings. My experience felt like I was always bundled up with outdated hospital policy based on outdated evidence that wasn't fit for making individualised decisions in the here and now. I ended up having an AMAZING VBAC, in huge part because of your book and the immense confidence and self-empowerment I derived from it! Any woman having a VBAC should connect with your book. Hospitals and birth support people should have your book as the first resource they offer to people looking to birth via VBAC!"

REFLECTION

Supporting women to be active in labour.

- Reflecting on the birth environment section of this chapter, how does the environment that you practice in impact women's labour and birth experience? Does it support being active in labour and upright birthing positions? How could you change the environment to support women better?

- Reflecting on the methods to remain active in labour section of this chapter, do you use any of these methods? How does your birth environment support the use of these methods? What methods do you want to learn more about?

- Reflecting on the use of CTG's during labour, if a woman approached you and asked for intermittent monitoring instead of a CTG, how would you approach this in a trauma-informed respectful way? What do you need to learn more about?

- Reflecting on the water immersion section of this chapter, how do you feel about supporting water immersion? How do women have access to water in your workplace?

"I can appreciate that OBs and midwives have no doubt seen and dealt with some horrible situations, and I am sure those memories haunt them. But please don't bring that into my birth. Don't project your fears onto me. Don't tell me that you've seen worst-case scenario, and that it happens more than I think. Don't dismiss the current and up-to-date research because of these experiences. And please don't disassociate from me and my birth for fear of the choices I've made."

Summary

Supporting women to be upright and active in labour, and to have access to water immersion and birth, is vital in creating a supportive birth environment that minimises stress, empowers women, and fosters positive relationships. There are challenges with this. Clinicians are often caught in a cycle of institutional pressures, work culture expectations, availability of resources and prescriptive guidelines (Ferguson et al., 2022). It can be difficult to step out of the cycle and put the woman back in the centre.

We need a paradigm shift in maternity care, moving away from a medicalised approach towards a more woman-centred model that respects women's autonomy, acknowledges their knowledge and preferences, and prioritises a safe and empowering birth experience.

CHAPTER 9

How to Support Women to Have a Gentle Caesarean

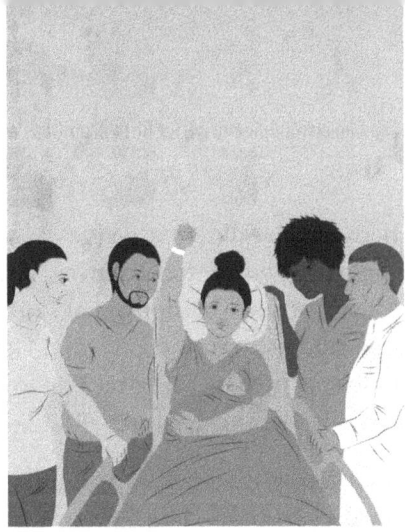

For many women, the thought of a caesarean section can evoke feelings of anxiety and disappointment. However, it's important to remember that a caesarean before or during labour can be a positive experience. By supporting women to actively participate in the planning of the caesarean, women can gain a greater sense of control and have a better birth after caesarean.

This chapter discusses how providers can support women to experience less trauma during a caesarean by considering options for a gentle caesarean.

The concept of a "gentle caesarean" emphasises a more woman-centred approach to caesareans. It involves creating a more supportive and personalised environment in the operating room, minimising unnecessary interventions, and prioritising the emotional and physical well-being of both mother and baby.

There are a few research studies that have explored the outcomes of using gentle caesarean methods. A study from Switzerland on 193 women explored the outcomes of an extended gentle caesarean protocol to their usual gentle caesarean protocol (Christoph et al., 2023). The extended protocol added the use of a transparent screen and maternal cutting of the umbilical cord, on top of the usual gentle protocol that included early intraoperative skin-to-skin contact, early breastfeeding, and avoidance of separation of woman and baby. Although there were no statistical differences in satisfaction, mother-to-child bond, and breastfeeding duration between the different gentle-caesarean styles, women who experienced the extended protocol showed preference for this style of caesarean in future births (Christoph et al., 2023). Similar findings were demonstrated in a studies from the USA and Germany that used a transparent screen, or lowering the screen and skin to skin compared to a standard caesarean protocol (Kram et al., 2021; Radtke et al., 2022).

A systematic review of II studies compared gentle caesarean to standard caesarean. The findings showed greater satisfaction of women in the gentle caesarean, alongside more skin-to-skin contact and initiation of breastfeeding, compared to the standard-caesarean method (Yuldasheva et al., 2023).

Having protocols is beneficial for the management of caesareans. However, I think there needs to be flexibility to ask the woman and her support team what a gentle caesarean looks like for them. There are a variety of aspects women may request for their gentle caesarean.

Creating a Calming Environment

+ Dimming the lights, playing soothing music, and minimising unnecessary noise can contribute to a more relaxed atmosphere. This may be particularly important for neurodiverse women and/ or partners who experience sensory overload, and for women who have a history of trauma.

Personalising the Environment

+ Playing music or sounds that are requested by the woman. This may encourage a culturally appropriate approach too. Introducing everyone in the room to the woman and support person.

Prioritising Skin-to-Skin Contact

+ Immediate skin-to-skin contact between the woman and baby is crucial for establishing early bonding and promoting breastfeeding. A previous caesarean with separation may have contributed to a traumatic experience.

Delayed Cord Clamping

- Allowing for delayed cord clamping provides the baby with additional blood and nutrients.

Minimising Separations

- Keeping the baby with the mother as much as possible, minimising unnecessary procedures, and allowing for extended breastfeeding opportunities in the operating room are essential. Measurements and weights can wait until they are in the postnatal ward.

Maternal-Assisted Caesarean

Techniques such as maternal-assisted caesarean, where the woman assists in delivering her baby, can empower women and enhance their sense of agency. In a maternal-assisted caesarean, the woman assists in the birth through reaching down with their hands in sterile gloves to lift out their baby (Tan et al., 2024). There is a growing number of obstetricians and hospitals that are offering a maternal-assisted caesarean, although there is limited research available at the time of writing.

In Australia, obstetrician, Dr. Natalie Elphinstone, started offering maternal-assisted caesareans in her private hospital in Victoria. In an article for the *Practising Midwife Australia*, Natalie indicated that it took a multidisciplinary approach to set up this caesarean style and explains how the process was undertaken (Elphinstone, 2023). Tan et al. (2024) has also provided a guide from the anaesthetists point of view of maternal-assisted caesarean.

Summary

While the availability of these practices may vary across hospitals, open communication between women and their health care providers is essential. Women should feel comfortable discussing their preferences and concerns regarding their caesarean births.

It's important to remember that every woman's experience is unique. The goal of a gentle caesarean is to create a more positive and empowering experience for each woman while ensuring the safety of both mother and baby. By working collaboratively with their health care providers, women can actively participate in their caesarean birth, and create more positive and memorable experiences.

REFLECTION

Supporting women to have a gentle caesarean.

- Reflecting on the gentle caesarean section described in this chapter, have you been involved in one? What was the experience like for you, the woman, and her family?
- If you don't have a gentle-caesarean protocol in your hospital, what would you need to do to set one up?
- How do you feel about a maternal-assisted caesarean? How would you assist a woman to have one at your hospital?

Have a look at the trauma-informed principles in

- Chapter 5. How can you incorporate these principles into how women experience a caesarean where you work?

"If an RCS is needed, discuss ways to make the experience more aligned with what mom would like. A gentler version without the trauma."

CHAPTER 10

Narratives From the Maternity Space

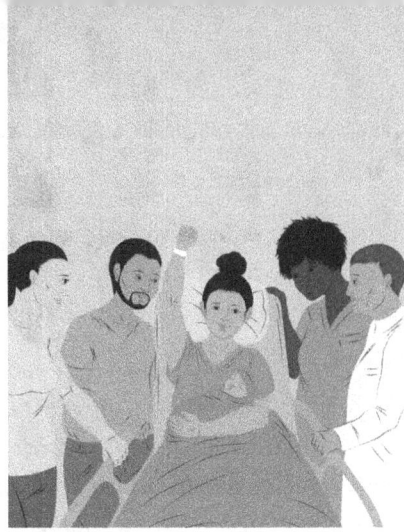

This chapter includes written stories from a variety of health care providers, and people in the maternity world, on how they support women to have a better birth after caesarean.

Nicole Garrat (Midwife) Reflection

Why do you think it is important to support women to have a better birth after caesarean?

We know that women's birth experiences shape their journeys into motherhood and with themselves. Their birth experiences can leave them feeling strong and empowered, or broken and mistrustful of their bodies. Also, many women wish to have more than 1 to 2 children, and the risk increases for each Lower Segment Caesarean Section.

What does a better birth after caesarean look like to you?

A birth where women's choices are heard AND respected. Where we choose women over policy. Where women have support to do what feels best for them, even if it is "not recommended" by policy.

How do you prepare women for a VBAC during pregnancy?

Discuss the woman's individual risk factors (e.g., multiple previous LSCS, short inter-pregnancy interval, high BMI, GDM etc). We talk about what "issues" will be raised by the hospital team before she even sees them. We talk about "risk" and what the real numbers look like. I don't shy away from the hard topics, such as how many babies *actually* die, what does an "adverse outcome" look like to her?

I encourage women to take notes to their appointments with the obstetric team—questions and notes relating to stats, and the evidence and papers those stats have come from.

> **It really annoys me that women need to come prepared with almost a PowerPoint presentation as to why they are willing, or not willing, to accept certain recommendations. But I have found these conversations go more smoothly, and the women feel less intimidated when they have hard stats in front of them, especially if they feel being put on the spot will make them feel flustered.*

How do you discuss with women who are planning a VBAC what a repeat caesarean may look like?

We talk about what she liked and didn't like with her previous caesarean. How can we make that better this time? We talk about what an unplanned caesarean in labour looks like (one where there is time to talk and make decisions), as opposed to a CAT 1, or even if she changes her mind and would like to book a planned caesarean. We talk about risks for next pregnancy, recovery, less likely to be supported for VBAC after 2 LSCS.

Is there a specific woman's better birth after caesarean that you remember? Why is that?

Woman had a VBAC after three previous caesareans, two of which were classical incisions. It was so memorable because everyone told her she couldn't do it—too dangerous, no one would support her, "just can't be done," to accept her history and try to make her next caesarean as "good as it could be."

Hx—G4P3—2 classical incisions, one LSCS

P1—baby born at 24 weeks and passed away a few days later.

P2—Unplanned caesarean due to spontaneous labour at 37 weeks (prior to booked date). Lost twin at 10 weeks, cervical shortening from 27 weeks. Started as LSCS, and then classical incision as she had been told there had been some scar dehiscence. She recalls being so frightened after first birth when doctors told her she "absolutely could not labour," and it was "very dangerous." When she went into spontaneous labour prior to her booked date, she literally turned up in a panic, still in her wet swimmers from getting out of the pool but was then left in a waiting room for hours while she contracted and literally thought "she would explode" due to all the fear around going into labour. After birth, she found out she had been about 6 cm dilated at time of caesarean.

P3—a booked section at 38+ that she felt so much grief over as she felt she "just had no choice." She was told original classical scar was "fine" and therefore LSCS was performed. She had certain wishes for that section that were not respected—delayed cord clamping, skin to skin in OT.

With her most recent pregnancy (baby #4), she started researching her options early. She was not opposed to a caesarean, but was adamant she wanted to know *all* her options. We discussed options being booked elective LSCS, awaiting spontaneous labour, and then accepting an LSCS, planning a VBAC (with a back-up plan if we needed to convert to LSCS). She was happy to accept repeat LSCS if there was a "true medical indication" for her or baby. She did not consider her previous uterine scars as a medical indication.

We looked at all her risk factors, including her age (over 35), number of previous caesareans (and the fact she had two classical incisions), and the short inter-pregnancy interval. We discussed what would be raised in her appointments with the OB team. We talked about the hospital VBAC policy, including IV access and CTG monitoring (she declined both).

We had a detailed record of understanding, after discussions with the OB team, and the woman agreed to moving to hospital as soon as labour started opposed to labouring at home for as long as possible before coming in.

We looked at resources on the "VBAC Facts" website, Special Scars Special Hope, Hazel Keedle's book, and listened to podcasts of women who had similar stories.

Their warnings that "your baby could die" really touched a nerve with her as her first baby DID die at 24 weeks after a classical incision caesarean. Therefore, she very much felt that LSCS being touted as a "cure" for death was overrated and untrue.

They tried to push LSCS, even using a maternal-assisted caesarean as an incentive. They wouldn't be able to offer that if it was an unplanned LSCS. They suggested she move her care to a hospital 40 minutes away that was "better equipped in case of an emergency". They suggested they could support her going into spontaneous labour, but then take her for LSCS if "labour is what was truly important to her". She stood her ground. When the time came for pushing, they wanted her to "get on the bed so they could give her a little bit of help (vacuum)." She declined. Her whole labour from start to finish was less than 3 hours, and her little girl was born in very few pushes.

SHE DID IT!!!!

> ** *I have included her own story below and I have shared everything with her permission*

If you have had a poor outcome of the mother or baby following a birth after caesarean, how did you cope with that and continue to support future women's birthing choices?

I can't think of an example where I have had a poor outcome. The only thing that comes to mind is how much more difficult the recovery can be for some women. Because of this, I don't sugar coat how a caesarean is major abdominal surgery. Doctors are very good at them, and do them often, but sometimes I feel this means we bypass the fact that it's a major surgery for both the woman and baby.

What advice would you give clinicians reading the book on how to support women to have a better birth after caesarean?

Firstly, it's not about YOU. It's about the woman and HER choices. You can support a woman safely and respectfully even if you don't agree with her choices. Listen to her. What is really important? Sometimes it's the little things (like being the first person to hold or touch her baby), or to feel her body go into labour naturally. Be solutions focussed. How can you negotiate on policies to meet her needs? How can you have discussions with other care providers to ensure respectful care? If you don't feel comfortable supporting her, then find someone who is because she will *feel* your uneasiness and you will derail her birth with your fears.

Nikki's Story

Little Fairy Blossom. I felt so much healing and growth during her pregnancy, I knew her birth was going to feel different for us.

I knew her birth was going to provide so much healing and light—whichever way it went.

Even though I could feel the healing, I was still unprepared for how much her birth and holding her would provide.

Everything happened so fast.

A 2-hour labour and she was in my arms.

My arms first.

I was told over and over by the hospital system that natural labour and vaginal delivery wasn't supported, recommended, or advised for me. That I was going against all policies and procedures. The hospital was extremely uncomfortable with my choices. To the point of recommending I try another hospital.

There were so many obstacles, challenges, and push backs, but with the support, guidance, love, and belief from Nicole, the amazingly supporting and loving medical team on the day, and Inca's intuitive knowing, she arrived safely, intervention and drug free.

Our first baby was rushed straight to NICU after an emergency caesarean. She was 6 days old when I got to hold her.

Our second baby, labelled an emergency caesarean, was delivered by a doctor, handed to a midwife and then handed to me.

Our third baby—a booked caesarean, as I was told this was all I was "allowed." So again, I had to wait to be handed my baby.

Our fourth baby, the first baby that I held first.

I got to scoop her up while her umbilical cord still connected us together.

I got to decide how I held her.

I got to decide how long her cord connected us.

She got to feel my touch first.

It might not sound like a big deal, but it was the biggest, most time standing still, monumentally healing moment.

Gail Colquhoun (Midwife) Reflection

Gail Colquhoun registered as a midwife in the NHS in Scotland in January 1998. 27 Years as a Midwife this year, and 4th Year as an Endorsed Midwife, Gail offers the full continuum of care that includes home-birthing and supporting VBAC/HBAC. Her midwifery practice is called The Nesting Hub Pty Ltd.

With the continued rise in intervention rates across labour and birth, and with the increase in birth-trauma rates reported too, as a Privately Practicing Endorsed Midwife in Sydney, I am receiving a steady increase in the number of enquiries from pregnant people keen to explore Vaginal Birth After Caesarean (VBAC) and/or Homebirth After Caesarean (HBAC). With the media coverage in recent times, in addition to the NSW Parliamentary Inquiry into Birth Trauma, it has come to the fore that those pregnant now wish more choice. They wish their voice to be heard, they wish respectful maternity care, and ultimately, they wish to be in full control of their labour and birth experience, and to support normal physiology as much as they can.

The private model of midwifery care that we as endorsed midwives provide support those choices, in offering continuity of midwifery care and home-birthing, with home-based midwifery care and support provided throughout pregnancy, labour, birth and then on, up until 6 weeks postpartum. Our clients remain at the centre of our model, and the control lies with them. With us as their health care providers, walking along-side them on their journey to birth and beyond, providing support, encouragement, respect and safe, evidence-based care, each step of the way.

Each day in life we live with risk, and we as midwives are appreciative that, in the birthing world, that risk can heighten or reduce depending on circumstance. Second by second, minute by minute, the landscape can change. We are ready to act whenever it does, and all whilst supporting our clients accordingly. In private practice, where we provide home-based care away from the hospital setting, it is imperative to manage that risk, for the safety and wellbeing of those in our care. Part of the risk management with those wishing to have a VBAC/HBAC, is having a clear understanding along with open and frank discussions about each aspect.

We acknowledge that surgical obstetric procedures carry risk such as infection, increased blood loss, potential damage to organs and of developing conditions, such as a deep vein thrombosis. In addition, a caesarean section also carries risks for the baby, such as respiratory distress syndrome (RDS), transient tachypnoea of the newborn (TTN), and potential trauma from instruments used during the caesarean. Therefore, in supporting those who choose our model of maternity care, and in our quest to reduce medicalisation, intervention, risk, adverse outcomes, and birth trauma, we support VBAC and HBAC (depending on circumstance) for those who wish to choose this option.

In considering a better birth after caesarean, it's important that women choose their maternity care provider carefully. I believe that this person should align with the clients' same thoughts and feelings, and to be respectful of their choices. As a homebirth midwife who provides continuity of care, I support normal physiology. I provide evidence-based midwifery care that enables informed choice and empowered decision-making. As private midwives, we allow the passage of time for labour and birth to physiologically unfold, in the most natural way possible. From the statistics held since The Nesting Hub began, the evidence is there that, supporting physiology and affording the body and baby the time to work together in harmony, the risks are reduced for birthing people and their babies. We know this to be true, having held a 0% emergency transfer rate up until now.

Supporting physiological birth at home allows the body to relax, and an uninterrupted flow of the body's natural oxytocin, our love hormone. Furthermore, when our clients feel safe, supported, cared for, empowered and undisturbed, it is more likely that a vaginal birth, and perhaps even a homebirth will occur, and in multiparous women with a previous difficult/traumatic birth, one hopes and believes that a better birth is achievable.

If a care provider has doubts about supporting their client's choices, then for me, that is a red flag, and it would be worthwhile for childbearing women to consider a different care provider, regardless of their stage of pregnancy. The care provider needs to believe in their client's ability to birth vaginally, and to be supportive as they step on each rung of the ladder, on their journey to birth and beyond.

In preparing clients for a VBAC/HBAC, I encourage clients to read the works by experienced midwife, academic, and VBAC researcher, Dr Hazel Keedle, and especially her fantastic book, *Birth After Caesarean: Your Journey to a Better Birth*. In addition, it is worthwhile exploring publications by the highly regarded Ina May Gaskin, Dr. Sara Wickham, Dr. Rachel Reed, Dr. Sarah Buckley, Dr. Melanie Jackson, Professor Hannah Dahlen, Jane Hardwicke Collings and Rhea Dempsey. As well as this, I encourage clients to read the evidence-based resource that is the VBAC Education Project, to listen to Podcasts such as The VBAC Link, VBAC Birth Stories, The Great Birth Rebellion, The Midwives Cauldron, and Australian Birth Stories, where evidence-based research and maternity care are discussed, and a plethora of interesting topics and journeys conveyed in each episode.

In addition, I suggest clients consider having the support of a labour and birth doula who focusses upon optimal maternal positioning (OMP), and for clients to engage with childbirth education programs to prepare them physically, mentally, emotionally, and spiritually for what lies ahead. Then for us, as midwives, to complement this with education, clinical care, support, positivity, and reassurance.

Furthermore, we would also discuss our client's personal circumstance, such as what led to their caesarean section previously. Had they laboured? And, if so, which stage in their labour did they reach before their caesarean section occurred? From my experience, those who have reached the active-labour stage previously have a higher chance of achieving a VBAC or HBAC.

However, having said that, I have also had clients who had not laboured before, but who achieved their VBAC or HBAC with determination and hard work from them, with good positioning for them and their baby, with a good flow of natural oxytocin, and with a supportive and caring partner and birth team. I never doubt a client's ability to birth their baby, and I am never concerned about the size of their baby either, contrary to what we see and hear in the media, and in the health care facilities that surround us. With a 0% post-dates induction rate held to date at The Nesting Hub, and with an exceptionally high vaginal birth rate too, this gives clients confidence, belief, positivity, and hope. However, I am also a realist, so clients are also made aware that occasionally VBACs and HBACs are not achieved, and labour and birth transfers can occur, despite great effort from birthing mothers, their babies, and from every-one in the birth team.

It is important to prepare pregnant people and couples for what a repeat caesarean section may look like, as we know that there is an increased risk of this manifesting, given the existing scar on their uterus. So as not to scare, it is imperative to highlight this, but also to reassure that the risk of rupture is still very small. The risk of a repeat caesarean section is also small, and as private midwives, we work hard to manage their labour accordingly, and safely. We monitor the intensity of the uterine activity experienced, to ensure that the uterus is not over-worked at each stage during labour, and our clients are also made aware to inform us if they experience pain around their uterine scar.

In addition, we assess their clinical wellness and their vital signs in labour. If a situation is arising, this will be identified in a timely manner, and swift action taken, if need be. Thankfully, caring for clients at home, where they feel most relaxed, and where we support physiological labour and birth, the uterus is under less strain.

In the hospital environment, where medicalisation and intervention rates are rising year upon year, I, of course, discuss the risk of uterine rupture at different gestations. Should a VBAC client wish to birth at home as an HBAC, then an obstetric consult is offered at 36-weeks gestation. I can join them for this visit, as their advocate and midwife, should they wish me to. If clients do not wish this consult to happen, then a full risk assessment is undertaken, and if I feel happy to continue on, as I have done with each VBAC or HBAC client so far, an individualised Record of Understanding, originally created by the Australian College of Midwives (ACM), is completed and signed by all parties. Following on from this, the care journey continues, and we prepare for our client's VBAC/HBAC. For our Nesting Hub clients who have chosen to transfer into the hospital at any stage, their midwife has stayed with them in the hospital, with unwavering support, advocacy, and encouragement throughout. It has been expressed that this has assisted in alleviating fears and anxieties surrounding their baby's entry into the world.

For our two AMAZING clients over the past 4 years who laboured long and hard before ending up with repeat caesarean sections, they felt empowered by labouring at home, they were more relaxed, they felt supported in their body's natural physiology, and they had belief in themselves and their birth team. They were also glad that their babies had the opportunity to move down the birth canal, exposing them to their mother's vaginal microbiota, dominated by Lactobacillus, Escherichia and Bacteroides, as they descended. With both, they reported their postpartum recovery was fast-tracked, and their breastmilk arrived in sooner than it had done following their previous caesarean section.

Over my past 27 years in midwifery, there have been many caesarean section journeys ... and a plethora of interesting stories too. However, one account that resonates most with me after all these years was a childbearing woman in the NHS in Scotland, who was pregnant with her 2nd baby. She had ended up with an emergency caesarean section in her 1st stage of labour last time, as her baby had become distressed, following an induction of labour. This time, she hoped for a VBAC. Her journey second time had become complex and convoluted, as she heartbreakingly developed breast cancer at 12 weeks gestation. She had wanted nothing more than to birth her baby through her vagina, and up into her arms. She, her partner, sister and I were fully on-board with making this happen, and through our continuity of midwifery care journey, and with each antenatal visit we shared, she felt more empowered and determined to make this vision a reality.

What we could not predict, in any way, was the escalation of her breast cancer, and when the safest time to birth would be for her and her baby. This wonderful woman really wanted a natural, physiological labour ... but, would her body and her baby respond and support this? It was anyone's guess. However, I always tell women to listen to their bodies, to believe that THEY CAN DO IT, and to tell their babies "when it's time," and that "they are ready." At 32 weeks gestation, THIS WAS THE TIME! ... as, the breast cancer had begun spreading.

During meditation, and while in a deep state of relaxation, this woman told her baby that it was time, and within 6 hours, her body went into spontaneous labour. How AMAZING are childbearing women, birthing people, and their babies? This phenomenal woman held her belief, she remained positive, she battled hard and ultimately, she achieved her VBAC. Then, in her postpartum, she continued her treatment pathway, and she beat breast cancer too.

I have been so fortunate in that I have not yet had a poor outcome of mother or baby following a birth after caesarean. However, I know colleagues who have. I know many devastating stories of families who have experienced this too. As continuity-of-care midwives, who provide care and support across the whole continuum, whatever the story, whatever the background ... we are there to listen, to hand-hold, to hug, to empathise, and to care. With the cascade of intervention, the rise in induction rates, and with the rise in caesarean section rates across NSW and beyond, we will strive to do all that we can to support normal physiology, and for our clients to remain front and centre. We will continue to protect and defend our clients and their choices going forward, as we continually endeavour to improve health outcomes for them, their babies, and for their families.

In an ideal world, and with regards to what advice I would give clinicians reading this book on how to support women to have a better birth after caesarean, I would like to see more respect, support, and appreciation given for our home-based private midwifery model of maternity care. I would like to see all Midwifery Group Practice (MGP) models of maternity care supporting all risk, and all offering labour and birth at home, if it is safe to do so.

Our statistics, as privately practicing endorsed midwives, reflect just how safe this model of care is, and how safe our clients and their babies are, with us as skilled, knowledgeable and experienced midwives. Birthing with a midwife is VERY DIFFERENT to those choosing to free birth. Therefore, it should never be treated, nor categorised in the same way as free birth. I am, of course, fully respectful of those who choose to free birth, and for some, they don't feel they have any other option. However, we as midwives attending homebirth are safe practitioners, skilled in identifying risk, managing risk, identifying deterioration, and then acting in a timely manner to provide effective, clinical care, and considering a transfer to hospital if circumstance warrants this. I would also like other health care professionals to be more accepting, and less fearful of us supporting VBAC/HBAC. It can be the most AMAZING journey to birth and beyond for these WONDERFUL people, and it can be such a healing birth for them too.

As a progressive move forward, akin to the many midwifery students that have gone before, we now have a medical student journeying alongside us on a client's journey to homebirth and beyond. It is hoped that this new exposure for medical students, who are our GPs, doctors, and potentially obstetricians of the future, will showcase this model of maternity care. It would be so heartwarming if it encouraged other medical professionals to explore our model of care, and to support VBAC and HBAC, now and into the future.

Midwife Gail

Claire Davison (Midwife) Reflection

Trusting women and birth: the key to supporting women to birth their babies after a caesarean.

Dedicated to Sally and Theresa, brave and exceptional midwives.

Dr. Clare Davison RM, RN, MPhil, PhD

I have been a midwife for 16 years, and have worked as a privately practising midwife, mainly attending homebirths since the beginning of my career. I have supported many women planning a VBAC after one, two, and three prior caesareans, and the majority of these women have had a physiological birth at home.

My midwifery philosophy guides my midwifery practice, which is the belief that birth is a normal physiological process that most women can achieve without intervention. I always knew I wanted to work in a continuity-of-care model. I tried to find a job in a midwifery-led setting in the public system, but at the time you needed a minimum of 3 years' experience to work in these settings. As I could not work in a midwifery-led setting, I accepted a graduate position in the hospital I trained at, started a Master of Philosophy, and tried to find a way to keep my passion alive. Luckily for me, I was able to transfer into the homebirth caseload setting very quickly after I graduated. Within a few months I was able to leave my graduate position in the hospital and become an apprentice to two wonderful midwives. This led to my ongoing passion for supporting women choosing to plan a vaginal birth after previously giving birth by caesarean section.

When I reflect on why I became so passionate about supporting women choosing a VBAC, a few key moments come to mind. Firstly, during my midwifery education, a woman was invited to tell her story. It was so powerful hearing about her journey and her eventually VBA2C. So much of this woman's story resonated with what I had seen: the lack of trust in women and birth, and the huge fear that seemed to prevail in the mainstream maternity system regarding VBAC.

The next key moment was pivotal, and led to me meeting my mentors, Sally and Theresa, and attending my first births at home. Just as she was about to leave a meeting with me, my academic supervisor received a text from one of the private midwives. "Do you want to be a back-up midwife for a VBAC in May?" she casually asked. My initial reaction was, "NO WAY! How could I support a VBAC? I didn't really know much, did I?"

However, after she left, I kept thinking about it. Could I be a back-up for this birth? Would this be a way to become the midwife I knew I could be? I texted my academic supervisor, could she give me the midwife's contact details? Maybe I could meet with the midwife to see what this would involve?

I arranged to go to the independent midwives' centre and meet the midwives. Sally Westbury, the midwife who needed the back-up midwife for May, was at a birth, so I didn't get to meet her that day, but I met Theresa Clifford. This meeting would change my life and career forever. I remember Theresa asking me why I thought I could be a homebirth midwife. I can't remember what I said during that initial meeting, but I must have said something right as she said she would speak to Sally and get back to me. Sally rang me later that day, and I arranged to meet her the following week where I would go with her to meet the women. If they liked me, maybe I would be able be a back-up midwife.

The next key event was the day I spent with Sally, and met the women. I met amazing strong women that day planning VBACs at home with Sally. They told me the stories of their previous births. One of the women, Cass, was planning her second VBAC. She gave me a DVD of her previous birth. When I got home, I watched it. It was the first time I had seen birth portrayed so positively. It was beautiful. I knew from talking to Cass that the birth had been long and hard, but SHE DID IT!!! At that moment, I knew beyond a doubt that I wanted to work with women like Cass, and midwives like Sally and Theresa.

The first three homebirths I attended as an "apprentice" back-up midwife were women having VBACs, and they all had straightforward physiological births. This makes it sound so boring. And to be honest, that is what it should be, but those births were magical. The midwife's watchful waiting as the woman took the lead, allowing her body to birth in the way she needed, supported by her family, the laughter, the tears, and celebration as the baby was born. No fuss or drama.

These reflections led to the reason for writing this contribution. What do women need from their midwife when they are planning their next birth after a caesarean?

My answer is very simple. The midwife needs to trust women and birth.

I believe the biggest barrier to women having VBACs is a lack of understanding of birth physiology. Most maternity care providers do not understand the physiology of birth. This is because most are not exposed to normal physiological birth. Historically, the midwife gained experience from attending births and knowledge was passed on through generations of midwives. Storytelling was used as a way of sharing knowledge, with both childbearing women and midwives sharing stories and women's ways of knowing. Previously, this knowledge was welcomed and accepted. Midwives trusted their gut instincts, intuition, embodied knowledge, and combined these ways of knowing with their practical skills and knowledge of the physiology of birth.

Nowadays, maternity care providers are constantly trying to make birth fit into a predefined picture of what birth should look like, but this is not how birth works. Constant checks on cervical dilation to assess labour progress are not only intrusive, but are not evidence-based and are irrelevant in a physiological birth. The cervix does not open in a linear way. Yes, it has to open to allow the baby to be born. But rather than focusing so much on the cervical dilation, we should be making sure that the woman is supported to work with her body.

The lack of trust in women and birth, and the medicalisation of birth that is based on risk-perception contributes to obstetricians and midwives using unnecessary medical or "just in case" interventions. This "just in case" care undermines women's belief and trust in their abilities and leads to midwives losing their trust and belief in birth.

A previous caesarean means that women have a small risk of the scar opening. I am not saying that this risk is not a big deal. I am saying this is a very small risk, and much smaller if we support the woman to work with her body rather than attach her to monitors and preform invasive examinations. Rather than telling the woman she can do it, this tells her that she can't.

Women have been birthing babies for millennia. Birth is a normal, natural function that is designed so well physiologically, that it rarely needs outside assistance. Contrary to popular belief, the medicalisation of childbirth in the Western world has not made birth safer. Research shows that often the high levels of intervention are not justified. In some cases, the high level of intervention is actually detrimental to birthing women. Midwives need to find that trust in birth and women's ability to do it. If you do not think she can do it, and the odds are already stacked against her. how will she believe she can?

I believe that most women can birth their babies without intervention. If there is a problem, it will present itself. Like the ripple in the still pond, if all you see is normal physiological birth in its wide range, then it is usually obvious when things start to move in an abnormal direction. I am there watchfully waiting and continually assessing, but without intervening unless I need to.

So, my advice for midwives wanting to support women to birth their babies vaginally after a previous caesarean is:

- Trust women.
- Trust birth.
- Understand physiology.
- Watchful waiting: learn the art of watching women carefully to work out what is happening in their labour.
- Support physiology; women and babies usually work it out together, but sometimes they need a bit of help.
- LISTEN to the women.

- Stop measuring labour in parameters that are not evidence-based (e.g., vaginal examinations or partograms).

- LISTEN to your intuition.

- Share birth stories with each other.

Being a midwife who supports home birth after caesarean (HBAC) can be extremely challenging at times. I found this out when in 2011 I was reported to the Australian Health Practitioner Regulation Agency (AHPRA) for the first time. There was a knock on the door at 5:30 pm on a Friday night, and I was handed a letter by a courier. I opened it and my life fell apart. My husband thought someone had died. He had never seen me so distressed.

Looking back now, it seems a bit weird that I was so absolutely devastated. But I had always prided myself on how good I was at my job. I was a first-class student at university, winning prizes and getting top marks in assignments and clinical practice. I transferred this into my midwifery care and took great pride in how I provided individualised, woman- centred, evidence-based safe care. I had been well respected when I worked in the system. In my naivety, I presumed this would continue now that I was a homebirth midwife. I was clueless!

Nowadays, I know so much more about the culture of midwifery in Australia. I am much more aware of the bullying of midwives and women who do not toe the party line. I joke that I have been set on fire so many times that I am almost fire resistant. But in the beginning, I was not blasé about it. I was devastated.

I had been reported to AHPRA by the Head of Midwifery at the tertiary hospital for unsafe practice. So, what had I done that was considered unsafe? I had provided care to a woman choosing to VBAC at home. I had recommended the woman see an obstetrician to discuss her choice, and I had booked her into a hospital. I thought I was demonstrating safe and collaborative care to a woman planning a VBAC.

The practitioner who completed the report had never seen the woman that the report was in response to. In fact, the woman had had an uncomplicated and speedy homebirth that morning. The report had been made a couple of weeks earlier, when the woman had attended an appointment to see an obstetrician at the hospital. Well played, Doctor! A report of unsafe practice is very serious. The onus was on me to prove I was safe, not on the person completing the notification to say how I was unsafe.

What followed were the most challenging times of my life, instead of being innocent until proven guilty, I had restrictions placed on my registration while the investigation took place. The investigation took over 2 years. This was very surprising as the woman had received care throughout her pregnancy, labour, and birth, and postnatally from me. The only other person who saw her was the obstetrician at 36 weeks for a routine appointment at the back up hospital.

I had provided AHPRA with all my documentation, so why did it take so long? Two years of hell, while I waited for the decision to be made. My ANF lawyer was amazing and very supportive, but we just had to wait for them to finish their investigations. Eventually, after 2 years, I received a letter, all it said was that we have found no evidence of unsafe practice. No apology. No recognition of what I had been through: the loss of earnings, self-worth, stress, and anxiety, and the toll it took on me and my family. Over the next couple of years, I received two more notifications for the same thing. Thankfully, both of these were dealt with much quicker as AHPRA appeared to recognise that homebirth midwives were being vexatiously reported.

For many, the experience of being reported gets the response that is intended. The midwife will leave practice as the stress and emotional toll is too much to bear. I understand this, as at times I also felt like walking away, but when it happened to me, I had to take a good hard look at myself and what I was doing, and it made me fight back.

I knew then that I was not unsafe. After being "cleared" of any wrong-doing, I am more confident in my practice now. If I get threatened with being reported, which unfortunately is still happening, I think go ahead. I am not scared of being reported anymore. I know I am providing safe, evidence-based midwifery care within my scope of practice. I know that the threat of reporting is at best a lack of understanding of the scope of midwifery practice, and at worst, a way to bully and control women and midwives. I am not going to be bullied anymore.

Vicki Hobbs (Doula) Reflection

Vicki is a doula and childbirth educator for over 20 years in Perth, Western Australia. Vicki also trains future doulas. Vicki can be found at www.backtobasicsbirthing.com.au

For over 20 years, I've worked as a doula, childbirth educator, and complementary therapist in Perth, Western Australia. My journey began as a remedial massage therapist specialising in pregnancy massage, where I often had pregnant women share their fears about childbirth. I found joy in helping ease their minds, offering tips on staying calm, working with their bodies, and trusting their instincts. Many of these women asked me to support them during labour, providing encouragement and massage to reduce discomfort and fear. Little did I know, I was already acting as an "unofficial" doula, and at that time I actually hadn't heard of the term "doula" as it wasn't commonly available in WA.

Inspired by these experiences, I trained as a childbirth educator and quickly realised how little many women and their partners knew about childbirth. Beyond the basics of pregnancy and labour, much of their knowledge came from dramatised TV portrayals of women screaming in pain. I wanted to change that narrative by focusing on educating and supporting first-time mums to prepare for physiological births, and reduce unnecessary interventions, particularly caesareans.

Over time, I noticed a growing trend: women seeking support for VBAC. These women often described their previous births as traumatising and clinical, and they longed for a more active, empowering role in their next birth. I dedicated my time in supporting more VBAC women, providing them with knowledge, confidence, and a voice in the birthing process.

When I began this work, VBAC-specific training was limited in Australia. I pursued international training, including a course from the UK, which left me wanting more. Then I discovered Jen Kamel's VBAC Facts in the US, and more recently Hazel Keedle's transformative work here in Australia. Their expertise reignited my passion and expanded my knowledge, despite the challenges of burnout and frustration with the maternity system's lack of individualised care.

Today, I run specific VBAC workshops to help women understand their bodies, the unpredictability of birth, and the importance of asking informed questions. I encourage them to advocate for themselves, much like a curious child who keeps asking "why." Just as importantly, I prepare couples for repeat caesareans, helping them feel more in control of the process.

Ultimately, my goal is to ensure women, and their partners feel heard, valued, and supported. Whether through education, guidance, or encouragement, I am committed to helping them have empowering, positive birth experiences that leave them feeling like active participants, not passive bystanders.

As a doula, two very different but deeply profound VBAC birth stories have left a lasting impact on me, and I'd like to share snippets of them with you.

The first story is about Mum A, who had a caesarean with her first child but was determined to have a different experience the second time. She felt unseen and unheard during her first birth, and this time, she was committed to putting her own wants and needs first. Though she wasn't entirely sure what she was looking for, she knew she wanted something better.

Living in a remote town, Mum A had to travel to Perth at 32 weeks to wait for the birth. We initially connected over the phone, and our conversation flowed effortlessly. She hired me as her doula, and it just felt right. That connection is so important when choosing a doula—you need to feel comfortable with the person who will be by your side during such vulnerable moments, and the doula must also feel that connection with the woman they are working with and supporting. Mum A was fun, super fit, and straightforward, and when we met in person, it felt like catching up with an old friend.

We spoke regularly, and I provided her with pregnancy massages, which became a time for deep, meaningful conversations about her birth plan, her needs, and the roles both I and her husband would play. She grew more confident with each conversation, and it was incredible to watch her happiness and self-assurance bloom.

As Christmas approached, Mum A went to an antenatal appointment, and everything was progressing beautifully. A few days later, she came to me for another massage. We talked about how relieved and excited she was, her determination to give birth vaginally, and how ready she felt to bring her baby into the world. That session was full of laughter and connection, and I felt such a strong bond with her.

During the massage, I let my hands flow intuitively, focusing on releasing tension and creating space for her baby. At the end, I guided her through a meditation—one of those rare moments where the words seemed to come from somewhere beyond me, as if I were channelling exactly what she needed to hear. I can't recall the words now, but I remember thinking, "this is something special." As I finished, quiet tears rolled down her cheeks. I sat beside her, wiped them away, and she smiled.

That moment felt sacred, a perfect expression of the trust and connection we had built together.

The following week, something happened that deeply affected me as a doula.

I remember it vividly. I was running a private hypnobirthing class for another VBAC couple at their home, and I was on call for Mum A. I had mentioned to Belinda that I needed to keep my phone close in case Mum A rang, and she was very understanding.

A couple of hours into the session, my phone rang. It was Mum A. Her voice was anxious as she explained that she'd been busy over the weekend attending family Christmas gatherings and couldn't recall feeling her baby move during that time and hadn't felt her baby move since then. I reassured her and suggested she go to the local hospital nearby. I told her to explain that she was from a remote town and ask if they could check the baby to ease her mind. She agreed and said she would call me back after.

Not long after, the phone rang again. This time, Mum A sounded distressed, her voice trembling, trying to control her sobbing. *"They've checked several times,"* she said, *"and they can't find a heartbeat. They want me to go to King Eddies."*

My heart sank. Without thinking, I instinctively said, *"It's okay."*

Her response was immediate and anguished: *"No, no, it's not fucking okay."*

Her words jolted me. I realized how thoughtless my response had been, and guilt swept over me. *"You're right,"* I said quickly. *"I'm so sorry. It's not okay. Let's get you to the hospital, and we'll go from there."*

When she arrived at the maternity hospital, the worst was confirmed: there was no heartbeat. Her baby was gone.

The heartbreak was immeasurable. Mum A now faced the unimaginable—starting labour and birthing her baby, knowing she would never take her baby home.

Her husband was hours away, travelling from their remote town to be with her. I couldn't stop thinking about how lonely and agonising that trip must have been for him, longing to be by her side, to hold her and grieve with her.

At the hospital, the blue teardrop sticker was placed on the door of the birth suite—a quiet symbol to everyone that this family was experiencing the loss of a baby. Those who entered the room did so with gentle compassion, their eyes and actions filled with respect and care.

One midwife stood out. She was extraordinary in her ability to support Mum A, gently reminding her that she was still birthing her baby—her beautiful, precious baby. She held Mum A, whispered words of encouragement, and helped her find moments of strength amidst the overwhelming grief.

The love and tenderness in that room was profound, even in the face of such tragedy. It was a moment that taught me how vital it is to simply be there, to hold space, to offer care, and to honour the deep love and grief that come with such loss.

In contrast, not everyone who entered the room showed the same level of compassion. One midwife, in particular, stood out for the wrong reasons. She came into the room several times, her demeanour cold and robotic, focused solely on completing administrative tasks and asking questions that just didn't seem appropriate in that moment. It felt as though she was ticking boxes, dotting the i's and crossing the t's, without any regard for the grieving woman in front of her. I remember thinking that she was not the right person for this role, not in these circumstances. Her presence felt out of place in such a sacred, emotionally charged moment.

Despite this, Mum A was absolutely magnificent during her labour. Everything she had learned about moving her body, breathing deeply, making noise, and staying calm, she put into action with incredible strength and determination.

I stayed by her side, rubbing her back and legs, holding her in moments when she needed comfort. We shared quiet laughter over silly things, trying to find lightness in the darkness, and we cried together, mourning the immense loss that surrounded her.

Mum A's energy shifted back and forth. At times, she was a lioness, strong, fierce, and powerful, fully immersed in the process of birthing her baby. Then, moments later, she would collapse into sobs, her body limp and wracked with grief. But through it all, she kept going.

Her love and determination was unwavering. She was committed to giving her baby the birth she had envisioned; a positive, calm, and loving experience, even in the face of such overwhelming heartbreak. Watching her navigate that journey was both devastating and deeply inspiring.

When her husband arrived, it was a tender moment of reunion—filled with grief but also love and support. It was time for me to step back and pass the baton, allowing them to hold space for each other. Quietly and respectfully, I slipped out of the room, giving them the privacy they needed to face this heartbreak together as a couple.

I found myself sitting in the chapel next door, a place I wouldn't normally go, as I'm not a religious person. Yet, in that moment, it felt natural, even comforting. I prayed to a higher power, asking for courage, strength, and love to surround Mum A, her husband, her family, and even myself. The stillness of the chapel allowed me to gather my thoughts and energy.

After what I think was about an hour, maybe more, a midwife came to let me know that Mum A was asking for me. I returned to the room, and it was clear that things had intensified. She needed more support: physically, emotionally, and mentally.

This was the moment when my "doula cape" went on, a visualisation I rely on during challenging births or difficult situations. The cape represents my ability to stay grounded and focused, no matter what is happening around me. Whether it's the push for unnecessary interventions, dismissive language toward a labouring woman, or other less-than-ideal circumstances, the cape helps me centre myself.

When I imagine putting it on, I feel a shift. It helps me breathe deeply, assess the situation with clarity, and provide calm, unwavering support. It's not about reacting with anger or aggression but about advocating for my clients with strength, respect, and positivity.

With the "cape" on, I was ready to be exactly what Mum A needed. I stayed by her side, giving her the reassurance and care she required to keep going.

And she kept going. With incredible strength and determination, she eventually roared her baby into the world, supported by the kind and compassionate midwife by her side. As the midwife carefully placed her perfectly formed, beautiful baby in her arms, there was a tenderness in every movement, protecting and honouring every part of this newborn in a deeply sacred way.

The moment of birth is etched into my mind forever, the undeniable reason for the loss of this precious baby. There was a true knot in the umbilical cord. From the placenta to the knot, the cord was thick, robust, and full of life-giving blood. But from the knot to the baby, it was pure white, empty. Nothing had been able to pass through to provide oxygen and nutrients.

Despite their grief, this mum and dad gazed through tears at their baby with profound love and pride.

At one point through her tears, Mum A looked at me and said, *"I did it, Vic. I got my VBAC. I know I can do it because I did it. I birthed my baby out of my vagina. I did it."*

Her words will stay with me for the rest of my life—a powerful reminder of her strength, her courage, and the love that carried her through even the darkest of moments for her to have a vaginal birth after caesarean.

It was a poignant reminder that where there is life, there is also death. As a doula, I felt deeply privileged to be part of this journey, supporting this couple through both the triumph of their VBAC, and the heartbreak of their loss.

The second VBAC story that deeply impacted me was that of Belinda, whom I had been sharing hypnobirthing with when I received the call from Mum A.

Belinda had experienced a caesarean for her first baby at a private hospital under the care of a private obstetrician. Throughout her pregnancy, she was repeatedly told that her baby was huge and that a vaginal birth was impossible. By the time she neared the end of her pregnancy, she felt as though giving birth vaginally would be physically impossible for her petite body, convinced that her baby would tear her apart.

At one point, her obstetrician explained that if the baby got stuck during birth, not only was there a risk of the baby dying, but she might also need a hysterectomy. Although the risk was low, the possibility lingered. He even shared a story from his training, where he had witnessed a birth where the baby got stuck, lost too much oxygen, and tragically passed away. Belinda was terrified by these possibilities.

Given the overwhelming fear of her body rupturing, the potential for the baby's death, and the possibility of needing a hysterectomy, it was understandable that Belinda opted for an elective caesarean. The fear simply outweighed all other considerations. However, Belinda went into spontaneous labour before her scheduled caesarean, which had been set for the day after her obstetrician returned from annual leave. Despite this, she was still taken to the theatre for a caesarean, with no discussion about the possibility of continuing with a physiological birth.

Her baby was a healthy, happy 3.81kg (8 lbs 4 oz), and at the time mum remembered thinking "hang on, wasn't he meant to be over 10 pounds?"

Working with this couple was an absolute privilege. I watched them transform from a place of fear to one of courage, and it was incredibly rewarding to see them find strength in their journey. This experience truly highlights why independent childbirth classes, the support of a doula, and a well-prepared mindset are essential, especially for those seeking a vaginal birth after a caesarean. Education, continuous care, support, and encouragement are the keys to overcoming obstacles, doubts, and blocks along the way.

To make a long story short, Belinda decided to book a different private obstetrician for her next birth, only to find that while this obstetrician was more tolerant of VBAC, they weren't truly supportive. So, she quickly switched again and found another obstetrician who seemed incredibly accommodating, accepting all the wishes from her birth plan. This obstetrician promised no induction, no stretch and sweeps, no vaginal exams, no cannula, no pain relief unless requested, no continuous monitoring. Basically, everything Belinda had hoped for. It felt almost too good to be true.

And, of course, it was.

This obstetrician, knowing she would be going on holiday and wouldn't be available around the due date, made it clear she wasn't truly invested in the birth. Instead, her backup would take over, and the responsibility of the birth would fall on someone else.

Belinda had chosen to have a private obstetrician in a public hospital, thinking that this would free her from the restrictive policies and procedures often found in private hospitals.

When Belinda went into labour at 40+2 weeks, I was there with her at home, holding her hand, reminding her to breathe, rubbing her tense muscles, and encouraging her to stay loose and flexible. We moved around, she hugged me, she connected with her baby, and focused on visualising the birth she wanted, not the things she feared. We had in depth conversations, we laughed, we cried (gosh, I feel like such a sook), and we positively anticipated a beautiful birth on that day.

If I could bottle the energy in that room, I'd be a millionaire. I've never seen a woman who once described herself as anxious, stressed, and fearful transform into a powerhouse of strength, determination, and sheer willpower. She grunted, she groaned, she made noise, and I marvelled as she channelled that energy to move her baby down.

It quickly became clear that she was ready to go to the hospital. When we arrived at the MFAU for assessment, the midwife called the replacement obstetrician to let him know that Belinda was there. After a few minutes, she returned and said that the obstetrician insisted on a vaginal exam, a cannula, and monitoring. Belinda, sticking to her birth plan, declined the vaginal exam and cannula. The midwife went back to the obstetrician, who insisted these procedures were non-negotiable or, "he was not stepping out of his front door." After several rounds of this back-and-forth, the obstetrician still refused to come in. Finally, Matt had enough. He told the midwife that his wife wasn't doing what she was told by this obstetrician. The midwife explained the obstetrician's policy but reminded them that Belinda had the right to refuse and to transfer care to become a public patient, which is exactly what she did.

I still beam with pride when I see Belinda share her birth story with others. She usually starts off by saying: *"I fired my private obstetrician while in active labour during my VBAC and it was the most liberating and empowering thing I could have done."*

The midwife then took Belinda to the birth suite.

Once again, I was in awe of Matt, watching him stand firm as a protector of his wife, their baby, and their birth space, ensuring that Belinda was treated with the respect and dignity she deserved. It was truly profound.

This is why it's so crucial for partners to be well-informed about what to expect, how to navigate the birth process, and their support, knowledge, and involvement are key in creating a positive birth experience.

During the birth, there were several challenges, many of which stemmed from midwives not listening to Belinda's wishes. She was spoken to and asked questions during surges, and at one point, I had to step in and request that they wait until her surge had passed before asking her questions.

However, there was one obstetrician who played a crucial role in making Belinda feel safe and calm. She was kind, spoke softly, and gently reassured Belinda. Before doing anything, she always asked for consent. Belinda later told me that she trusted this woman. Reflecting on her birth, Belinda said, "She was the only obstetrician who showed me respect and support that day."

Once Belinda felt safe, she described the sensation of her body "opening up." She felt a "burning" sensation around her perineum, but it wasn't painful. It gave her awareness of her body stretching and opening to allow her baby to emerge.

Baby Leilani was born at 40+2 and she weighed 3.91kg! Yes, that's right. She was exactly 100g BIGGER than Belinda's first born!!!

Belinda shared, *"It was amazing to feel my body opening up. Baby's head was out. Another strong wave, and baby's body slid out—the best feeling in the world. The release was instant. I grabbed my baby onto my chest, and she was calm, but not crying, only little grunts. I cried tears of joy. Everyone in the room cheered and cried. Matt kissed me and told me how proud he was of me, and I felt a love for him like no other. I cried happy, proud tears. Vicki cried and hugged me."*

One part of this VBAC that always makes me laugh happened not long after the birth and Belinda while holding her baby on her chest, suddenly did a fist pump into the air and shouted at the top of her lungs, *"Fuck you, (Obstetrician's name),"* which was aimed at the obstetrician who wouldn't step out of his front door unless she followed his rules.

Then, looking at me, she smiled through her tears and said, *"I did it! I gave birth out of my vagina. I got my VBAC!"*

Belinda reflecting on her birth says:

> *I still feel like a warrior. I still feel on top of the world. Not only did I achieve the birth my heart so deeply desired. I have a closer bond and love for my husband like no other, and I have gained a very special friend, our doula Vicki, for life. I will be forever grateful to her for being the backbone to my success. I will be forever grateful for coming across hypnobirthing and the tools and techniques we learnt together for birth that we can use for the rest of our lives. Not only did I get an amazing birth, but I feel like it has changed my life. My outlook on a whole lot of things has changed. I can't recommend enough how important it is to educate yourself and to have a great support network around you. If I can do it, so can you!"*

No more words needed.

These two VBAC stories, though vastly different in their journeys, highlight the profound strength, resilience, and courage of women in the face of adversity. Whether it was navigating the heart-wrenching loss of a baby or fighting through the fear and doubts that come with a previous traumatic birth, these mums each demonstrated an unwavering determination to take control of their births, advocate for their bodies, and, ultimately, achieve the birth they had always dreamed of. Their stories remind me of the deep importance of trust, support, and respect in the birthing process, and the transformative power of education, compassion, and a supportive birth team. Being part of these journeys was a privilege, and it's a constant reminder that as doulas, we are there not only for the birth of a baby but for the birth of a mother, a partner, and a family.

Katelyn Commerford (Doula) Reflection

Katelyn is a doula and NBAC guide working in Sydney for over two years.

Why do you think it is important to support women to have a better birth after caesarean?

The research tells us that women who have experienced a prior caesarean birth also experience higher rates of trauma. Birth is a transformational experience, and we owe it to these women to support them to have the most positive experience they can. Just as I believe we should be supporting each and every woman in our care to experience the best birth for them that we can.

What does a better birth after caesarean look like to you?

It's often vaginal, but not exclusively. More so the things that seem to matter have been whether she was truly supported in what she wanted, whether she felt she was able to give it everything she had, whether she felt she was in control of what happened to her, and was listened to when she expressed her wants and needs. It's whether she was treated as the most important person in her birth as opposed to a passive passenger in the process. The other crucial element has been no separation of mothers and babies where a caesarean pathway was taken. The importance of this cannot be underestimated.

How do you prepare women for a VBAC during pregnancy?

I spend a lot of time listening to their prior experiences and hearing their fears and their worries. We work on birth mapping to cover as many possible curveballs, and what these different pathways could look like, which gives her a sense of control. We talk about all the different options available for her labour. I usually lend them a copy of *Birth After Caesarean* to read through, as well.

We spend a lot of time preparing for circumstances that we know will be triggering, usually things that they found traumatic in their prior births, so that we get ahead of them as early as possible. To use a Keedle analogy, we try to do the weeding well ahead of the birth. The women that I support planning a VBAC are often wanting to go for an unmedicated birth, and so we also work on pain management tools and techniques, go over birth and hormonal physiology to understand their bodies in labour, and discuss hospital guidelines and how that will influence the recommendations made to them in labour and birth and compare that to what they actually want from their care so they know what conversation to have with their clinicians ahead of time.

How do you discuss with women who are planning a VBAC what a repeat caesarean may look like?

It's a critical part of the birth mapping process, and I make that very clear from the outset. I'm quite sensitive to the experiences they've previously had, and we approach the topic gently, but go over many of the different options for caesarean sections. We talk through all the various things they can ask for. I learn from them what are absolutely crucial requests in a repeat caesarean, and what things would be nice-to-haves if it works out, as well as what parts don't really bother them. I know which hospitals around me put their foot down at certain things, and I help to prepare them for the possibility of not having more than a minute of delayed cord clamping, for example, or not getting a second support person in the theatre. We talk about their rights when it comes to having their baby separated from them, and what they can do and say in the moment, as well as giving the partners advocacy tools for these possible moments as well.

Every woman I've supported for a planned VBAC has had a caesarean pathway map that was unique to them and their needs. I think that really demonstrates how crucial it is to treat each woman as an individual in her care, as well.

Is there a specific woman's better birth after caesarean that you remember? Why is that?

I can remember each woman's better birth after caesarean that I've supported. I'm lucky, as a doula, I choose my workload, and I keep to a very light caseload. The very first birth I supported was a woman planning a VBA2C, and she had had two traumatic inductions that were over practically before they began. Her VBA2C labour turned into a repeat caesarean about 36 hours in after a long 12 hours with no observable changes. I was devastated for her. I worried about how she would feel, but when I saw her a couple of days postnatally (after sneaking into the postnatal ward briefly after she got out of recovery), she was glowing. She was overjoyed to have been given the opportunity to really experience labour, and to leave no stone unturned in pursuing her VBAC. She had pushed back on a repeat caesarean multiple times during her labour until she felt like she had done it all, and to her, it was truly a better birth after caesarean.

One of my favourite things in the world is watching a woman who was previously told her body failed her push her baby out, and pull them to her chest and proclaim, "I did it." The reclamation in those moments is so powerful, and the healing of so many unhelpful and untruthful beliefs she has held about herself. You watch it all fall away, and so often, you know how powerful her preparation for this moment has been.

If you have had a poor outcome of the mother or baby following a birth after caesarean, how did you cope with that and continue to support future women's birthing choices?

Another woman's VBAC that will stay with me forever was a woman birthing at home after a caesarean. She had an epic labour with a suspected posterior baby, who it seemed had finally made her rotation to come on through, but the woman's contractions were spaced 10 minutes apart. It was coming up to sunrise, and she was utterly exhausted. We set her up on the bed so that she could sleep between contractions, and then when one would come, she would shift her leg and roar, pushing beautifully, and then fall promptly back to sleep. This went on, breaking all the rules of what a labour "should" look like, but with mum and bub both well, and baby coming further and further down with each push, we trusted the woman's body was doing what it needed.

We let her get the rest, and once baby's head was on view between contractions, we helped her back up into the pool where gravity and consciousness got her moving very quickly from there. She cried, and so did I, as she felt her baby's head leave her body. She scooped her baby up onto her chest and sobbed. Every person in that room believed in her, and with no other signs of concern, simply trusted her body and baby to do what they needed. It was an incredibly powerful birth.

They transferred to hospital a few hours postpartum based on some strange and concerning symptoms the baby had, and what they eventually learned was that their baby has a congenital condition. It was not something that could have been diagnosed or prevented in pregnancy at all, not something instigated by her birth, just one of those unpredictable and devastating anomalies. It meant her postpartum experience was not what she had planned for in the slightest. She confided in me that she didn't know how she could have gotten through it if she'd had another traumatic birth. The power of her birth gave her strength to keep going through a hugely tumultuous and worrying time. And that is a testament to why it's so important to support women to have a better birth after caesarean.

What advice would you give clinicians reading the book on how to support women to have a better birth after caesarean?

I think it is truly simple: listen to the women. Counsel them on risks and benefits, yes (but use the evidence). Provide recommendations where appropriate, yes, but ultimately support what the woman wants to do. And if you can't, if you don't feel comfortable or your biases are too strong, you have an ethical duty to refer that woman to someone who can support them.

Build up their confidence in their bodies and their ability to birth and put them at the centre of their pregnancy and birth experience. Remember that no one is more invested in the safety of their baby than its mother. Take your cues from her. Be her biggest cheerleader and support her to give it everything she wants to give it.

Push the boundaries of what is standard procedure in your institution; if a woman's birth turns to a caesarean in the middle of the night, what can you do to ensure that mother and baby are not separated? Remind yourself that the guidelines are for you to make recommendations, not laws for the women to follow. Allow them an opportunity to decline recommendations if that's what feels right for them. If they never knew they could say no, it wasn't consent in the first place. At the end of the day, it all comes back to the same first point: listen to the women and really hear them.

Hazel Keedle (Midwife) Reflection

I wrote the reflection below following Sasha's VBA2C at home where I was her midwife. Sasha shared her birth story in my first book, Birth after Caesarean, and has given permission for me to use her name in this reflection.

Lady Justice, holding balanced scales, a sword and blindfolded, is known as a figurative personification of the moral force in justice and originates from both Greek and Roman mythology. The image for me though is more akin to midwifery, and I have often used this imagery when discussing my role as a midwife to women planning to homebirth. Although I am usually only referring to this in antenatal discussions, I acutely felt the importance and relevance of this during a very recent homebirth. This may seem strange and suggest to you that I see myself as the "strong arm of the law." Far from it as I describe the fine balance of knowledge, reasoning, empathy, and support the midwife requires when supporting women in the home.

I find this more pertinent in the homebirth setting than I do in any other midwifery setting I have worked in due to the completeness and dependence of the midwifery role to herself and to just one other midwife (if they get there in time). There is no red buzzer to press, and then work as a team in an emergency scenario, and no senior professionals to come in and override your decisions. You are it, that continuity of carer, the trusted one, and ultimately the responsible one.

My client, Sasha, was one I knew well. Pregnant for the third time, I had been on her pregnancy and VBAC journey before, but it didn't go to plan and was a repeat emergency caesarean after wishing for a HBAC. I had been very disappointed for Sasha at the time, but logically felt that as the reason for caesarean was so similar to the first, then maybe that was how it was for her. Big babies, petite woman, long labours, little descent, caesarean. I was worried that this had broken our midwife–woman relationship and hoped she would be able to find peace and acceptance at some point. Eighteen months later, I was so happy to hear from her and find out she was pregnant again.

Sasha's first hurdle was deciding on where or who she would see for her antenatal care because she was well aware that her local hospital wasn't supportive of her wishes for a VBAC after two previous caesareans (VBA2C). Although I had moved since the last pregnancy, and was taking few clients due to my new position, I did offer her my midwifery services for appointments, and as support in the hospital, if she wished.

As the pregnancy advanced, Sasha and her partner increasingly wished to labour at home for as long as possible, and hope for a VBA2C in the hospital if possible. Appointments were had at the hospital, as required, and then continued with myself. Sasha was aware about VBAC from her last pregnancy. She had read and absorbed everything she possibly could, so this pregnancy was more relaxed and chatty, plus she was busy with two kids and her family business.

After about a week of on/off contractions, Sasha called me on a weekend night just after midnight. The contractions had woken her, and felt stronger, and now regular around 4 mins apart. I set off to her home, and a few hours after I was there, I called my second midwife.

Sasha has labours that, at times, appear that she is about to push, and at times settle, and she can rest a bit, typical undisturbed long labours. She is amazing during a contraction. She finds her rhythm, and breathes or moans away, and always uses her body in movement. You ask her to get out of the pool to walk, and she does. Lunge on the stairs? No problem! Just wonderful to watch. But they are long and everyone gets tired, especially the labouring woman.

Emotions were raw and exposed, and her support team unfailing in love and encouragement. As labour wore her down, I realised she had no belief that she could do this, and no-one there could guarantee her the outcome either. It was really tough on her, and challenging for me.

A woman having a VBA2C has similar uterine rupture rates than women having a VBAC after one caesarean. But somehow, that doesn't translate into clinical practice. Maybe because the woman in front of you isn't a statistic, but a real woman who has had two previous caesareans, and as a clinician you are just so much more risk aware.

Reasoning influences your thoughts. Well, she has had two, the chances are so small! The "what if's" seem bigger. What if the uterus ruptures? Will a long labour influence this? Would I spot the rupture? Would I be too late? Threats loom ahead, what if I get reported? I had just come out of the national homebirth midwife audit, and although I passed, the process was intrusive and unsettling. I didn't want to invite this presence back through being reported. The doubts and fears can become crippling; they mustn't be dismissed completely, but they must be kept in check.

That is where Lady Justice comes in for me, as she did during Sasha's labour. I was Lady Justice. In my hands were the scales: one carrying the woman, one carrying her baby. The scales were in balance if my clinical judgement felt they were both well, tipped either way if one was not. My observations and senses were used to judge this. From basic midwifery skills of maternal observations, and intermittent auscultation, to supporting through emotional moments of doubt help me see how the scales are balancing. If both are balanced, we can carry on.

The sword is my role as her advocate. Such an important role requires a strong object. Not a weapon that I threaten or attack with, but one that I carefully hold beside myself and touch it's handle when I need the strength to speak up and speak out. When I am entrusted as an advocate, I not only remind women of their voice amongst other practitioners, but remind them of their own wishes. At times, I gently reminded Sasha of what she wanted to do as she was doubting her ability, and crying, "who am I trying to kid?"

And then the blindfold. Well, this one is to remind me to feel. Not to just see what my eyes can see, but to see beyond, and to feel within. It's empathy and checking in. How is the woman feeling and why? How are the support people feeling and why? How do I feel and why?

Are my fears bubbling over into my words and actions? Take a moment, reflect, adjust, and carry on.

Through Sasha's long labour, I walked as Lady Justice, my mind constantly checking in on the scales and forever trying to rationalise whilst trying to read all the emotions around and within me. It's exhausting, but it's what we do.

Although the vaginal examinations were pretty inconclusive, and not particularly helpful in "assessing progress," they did indicate a large bulging forewaters that once released would most likely bring that baby down. How far was uncertain and new territory. Finally, they spontaneously ruptured, and shortly afterwards, Sasha displayed behavioural and physiological signs of second stage.

This had never happened to Sasha before, and the new sensations were scary and uncertain. At one point, I suggested she reach inside to see what she could feel. I suspected (and hoped) that within reach was the head, and I was right, she felt it. I thought this would be the moment she believed she could do it, but it wasn't.

Though it was helpful for her to feel how the head had come closer. Doubt was still present, and Sasha feared that the baby would now get stuck. Encouragement and praise was oozing from everyone there, and she kept going. In just under 2 hours, the unbelievable happened. In the birthing pool by herself, she reached down and lifted her baby out of the water and onto her chest. The moment had come despite all her doubts and fears and disbelief. She did it!

What did I learn? So much! Sasha had her VBA2C even though she never thought she could until her baby's head was born. Most importantly for me was the recognition of support. I couldn't believe she would have a VBAC, but that wasn't necessary. By channelling Lady Justice, keeping the scales balanced, the sword by my side, and the blindfold on to tap into more than the eyes can see, I was able to give Sasha the opportunity to try. Strip away the constricting policies and guidelines, and there we find Lady Justice, or more accurately, Lady Midwife.

Reflections from Indonesia

There are now four reflections from midwives in Indonesia. I would like to thank Erni Rosita Dewi and Ruang Bidan. Erni translated the reflections from Indonesian to English. Indonesia holds a special part in my heart, and I am thrilled to include their reflections in my book.

Alfia Handayani Hatta (Midwife) Reflection

Alfia is a clinical midwife of 13 years, working in a Health Centre in South Sulawesi Province, Indonesia.

Why do you think it is important to support women to have a better birth after caesarean?

Providing women with the opportunity to make informed choices about their birth experience empowers them to take control of their own health care decisions. VBAC provides an opportunity for women to actively participate in the birthing process and potentially have a different and more positive experience compared to a caesarean section. In addition, vaginal delivery generally has a shorter recovery time and fewer complications compared to caesarean delivery. Supporting VBAC can reduce the risk of surgical complications, such as infection, blood loss, and longer hospital stays, thereby speeding the mother's physical recovery. This has happened a lot in my current place of duty. Many mothers who give birth by CS experience CS wound infections.

Multiple caesarean sections may increase the risks associated with subsequent pregnancies, such as uterine rupture, placental complications, and the need for additional surgical intervention. Supporting VBAC allows women to avoid these risks and have more options for future pregnancies.

VBAC is often associated with lower health care costs compared to repeat caesarean section due to shorter hospital stays and lower surgical costs. Supporting VBAC can contribute to a more cost-effective health care delivery system. Even though the costs of giving birth are covered by the government, either through BPJS Health or Jampersal insurance, the costs for the caring family are not covered. Because post-CS care takes longer than vaginal delivery, CS costs more than vaginal delivery.

What does a better birth after caesarean look like to you?

Women are empowered with comprehensive information about their birthing options, including the risks and benefits of VBAC (Vaginal Birth After Caesarean) versus repeat caesarean section. They can discuss their preferences, concerns, and health history with health care providers to make decisions that align with their values and goals.

Women receive personalized care and support throughout the birthing process. This includes access to health care professionals experienced in supporting VBAC, as well as emotional support to overcome fears or anxieties related to previous caesarean experiences.

Physiological Support for Vaginal Delivery: Women are provided with optimal support to facilitate successful vaginal delivery. This may involve techniques, such as induction or augmentation of labour, monitoring for signs of uterine rupture, and access to pain management options tailored to their preferences and comfort.

The birthing process is allowed to proceed as naturally as possible, with minimal medical intervention unless necessary for the health and safety of mother and baby. This may involve avoiding unnecessary caesarean sections and interventions that may increase the risk of complications or interfere with the progress of labour.

Women feel supported, respected, and empowered throughout their birthing experience, whatever the outcome. Whether they successfully achieve a VBAC or require a repeat caesarean section, they feel heard, valued, and involved in decisions regarding their care. The ultimate goal is to achieve the best outcomes for mother and baby, including optimal physical health, emotional well-being and bonding. This may involve proactive management of any complications that arise during labour, as well as postnatal support for recovery and adjustment.

So, in my opinion a better birth after caesarean section involves informed-decision making, personalized care and support, physiological support for normal birth, reduced medical intervention, a positive birth experience, and a healthy outcome for mother and baby. It prioritizes the holistic well-being of women and their families, respecting their autonomy and preferences while ensuring safe and evidence-based care.

How do you prepare women for a VBAC during pregnancy?

Carrying out an integrated ANC examination to detect early complications that may occur during pregnancy and childbirth. Apart from that, we, the community-health-centre midwives, are carrying out a government program, namely holding classes for pregnant women accompanied by pregnancy counselling, although it has not been running optimally to date.

Education for pregnant women and their families is also really needed because many pregnant women choose to undergo CS because they are afraid of feeling pain during childbirth, whether because of the trauma of a previous birth, or because they received inaccurate information from relatives. Mothers who fail at induction, and end up having a caesarean usually prefer a planned caesarean even though currently the pregnancy has a chance of a normal birth. The lack of optimal delivery services available at health facilities such as community health centres causes a lot of trauma to pregnant women.

How do you discuss with women who are planning a VBAC what a repeat caesarean may look like?

During pregnancy, I will inform you about the possibilities that will occur during childbirth. And I will do it repeatedly with different material at each ANC visit, or when attending classes for pregnant women. Pregnant women who are planning a VBAC will be as prepared as possible, both physically and mentally. I will inform you that even though the pregnancy is currently progressing normally and well, the mother and baby are healthy and safe for spontaneous labour. But there is still a possibility that the labour will end in CS. Because there are many maternal factors that influence the mother's pregnancy and childbirth. We humans can only try and pray, and the rest is left to the creator. What's wrong with trying to give the best for us and our children?

Mental support is really needed for this, not only from the mother herself or from the midwife, but from the family and close relatives of the pregnant woman. As much education as possible should be given to the pregnant woman's husband and family. At the very least, mothers and husbands should get information about VBAC including its potential failure.

Is there a specific woman's better birth after caesarean that you remember? Why is that?

Yes, there is. Because I work in remote areas on the islands, the personal hygiene of my mothers and families is very poor, causing many surgical wounds to become infected. So, it is not uncommon for re-stitching to be done in the hospital. Not only does the mother feel pain for a long time, but it also takes a long time so that the mother and family cannot work immediately after giving birth. This has an economic impact on the mother's family. Newborn babies will also receive less-than-optimal care. Mothers and families focus on healing surgical wounds so that breastfeeding for babies is reduced.

With the myth developing in society that post-CS mothers should not move much, the mother's mobilization is reduced resulting in longer healing of CS wounds. It can even reach 6 months or more. While mothers who give birth spontaneously/vaginally do not need a long time after giving birth. It is not uncommon for mothers who have given birth normally to immediately carry out their normal activities the day after giving birth.

The last case I encountered was a 25-year-old mother with her first child premature due to rupture of membranes, and a 6-year gap between pregnancies. The second pregnancy, both mother and baby were healthy. The birth was normal at the community health centre where I work. Unfortunately, the mother was traumatized by the CS because an infection occurred from the wound so it had to be re-stitched on the 16th day after surgery. Thank God, the second child was birthed spontaneously, and the day after giving birth, the mother was able to carry out household activities. Currently, the baby is 2 years old, and the mother is now pregnant with her 3rd child.

If you have had a poor outcome of the mother or baby following a birth after caesarean, how did you cope with that and continue to support future women's birthing choices?

I will provide education regarding problems that occur in mothers and babies, the possible causes of these problems, and how to overcome them. The education I provide uses language that is easy for mothers and families to understand. If it is possible that the mother will become pregnant again, the problem she is facing now should be prevented as much as possible. Monitoring during pregnancy greatly influences the health of the mother and baby. Apart from that, the cooperative attitude of the mother and family towards the education provided also has a big influence. I hope that with this, mothers will no longer be traumatized by being pregnant and giving birth, so that the process of pregnancy and giving birth can be enjoyable.

What advice would you give clinicians reading the book on how to support women to have a better birth after caesarean?

For clinicians who read this book, keep your knowledge up to date. Continue to learn about the latest evidence-based practices, guidelines, and research regarding VBAC (Vaginal Birth After Caesarean) and caesarean section. Stay informed about best practices in supporting women through the birthing process, including strategies to promote successful VBAC. As well as providing comprehensive information to women regarding their birthing options, including the risks and benefits of VBAC compared to repeat caesarean section. Make sure women understand the factors that may influence their eligibility for a VBAC, such as a history of previous caesarean sections, the type of scar on the uterus, and any associated medical conditions. Support women in achieving a successful vaginal birth by encouraging the physiological process and minimizing unnecessary interventions.

When promoting VBAC, also be prepared to manage potential complications that may arise during labour. Maintain vigilance for signs of uterine rupture or other emergencies and implement protocols for timely intervention and transfer to higher level care if necessary. All of this together effectively supports women to have better births after caesarean section, promoting positive outcomes for mothers and babies while respecting women's autonomy and preferences in the birthing process.

Azmiatun Nisa (Midwife) Reflection

Azmiatun is a community midwife of 2 years, working in a health centre in West Java, Indonesia.

Why do you think it is important to support women to have a better birth after caesarean?

Looking at the long-term side effects of a caesarean section and returning to a woman's natural state. That a woman's body has been designed by God to be able to conceive, give birth, and breastfeed. That is a physiological thing, which we need to optimize.

What does a better birth after caesarean look like to you?

If you meet the requirements, choose to give birth vaginally.

How do you prepare women for a VBAC during pregnancy?

Provide education to pregnant women and their families about VBAC, provide a journal of what activities need to be prepared to achieve a VBAC birth, such as looking for a provider and place of birth that is pro VBAC, breathing exercises, physical exercise, and mindfulness, not forgetting the family environment that supports the mother's choice to VBAC.

How do you discuss with women who are planning a VBAC what a repeat caesarean may look like?

Carrying out interpersonal communication, apart from that, as a village midwife, you can also do home visits, so that you can explain the type of birth that the mother chooses and the risks not only to her husband, but also to family members who live in the same house as her.

Is there a specific woman's better birth after caesarean that you remember? Why is that?

Never, because most of my patients with a history of CS prefer to give birth via CS.

If you have had a poor outcome of the mother or baby following a birth after caesarean, how did you cope with that and continue to support future women's birthing choices?

In accordance with existing procedures at the community health centre, namely carrying out home visits by village midwives to monitor the condition of the mother and baby. If the condition worsens, a referral will be made to a more adequate health facility (hospital) by first consulting a doctor at the health centre. Take a personal approach to ask about previous birth experiences, and provide education about the advantages and disadvantages of the birth method that will be chosen in the future.

What advice would you give clinicians reading the book on how to support women to have a better birth after caesarean?

It is recommended that clinicians, particularly those employed in government-owned basic services (Puskesmas), gradually modify their approach and service delivery flow. This will allow mothers who have previously given birth vaginally to continue doing so.

Ferninda Sagita Ramadani (Midwife) Reflection

Ferninda is a midwife of 4 years working in private practice in Indonesia.

Why do you think it is important to support women to have a better birth after caesarean?

Because for women who get the best support from their environment, especially from their midwives, the outcome will be better than before. Not only medical outcomes but psychological outcomes also. Then, the outcome will make their nurture process better.

What does a better birth after caesarean look like to you?

The birth process is chosen mindfully by the women. It means they know why they got the caesarean in their past birth process. They know how to cope with the uncommon things which will come to their process.

+ The women have the right and power in their process.

◆ The women have a bigger involvement in their birth process, not depending on their provider.

How do you prepare women for a VBAC during pregnancy?

The long process, actually, first my team and I must know what the biggest motivation of the VBAC. Then, we have several discussions about:

1. Do they have trauma in their past birth process?

2. Do they get clear information about the reason "why they got caesar?"

3. What have they done to prevent the prognosis that will lead to caesarean birth again?

4. What have they done in VBAC preparation during their pregnancy?

5. We discuss nutrition, lab examination, physical, psychological, spiritual, and social support preparation.

6. We do prenatal yoga.

7. We discuss their birth plan and the worst-case scenario.

How do you discuss with women who are planning a VBAC what a repeat caesarean may look like?

We provide the information about their condition which can suddenly lead to repeat caesarean. We agree that if a repeat caesarean happens, it doesn't mean they are failed. They will experience a better caesarean because they have learned better and know their body and babies' needs mindfully. Never give a judgement statement to the women, say that, "The baby chooses his/her own process about how they will be given birth."

Is there a specific woman's better birth after caesarean that you remember? Why is that?

Yes, I remember that she had a traumatic caesarean in her previous birth. After several hours, her baby was gone. So, it made the mother feel so traumatised and scared in her second pregnancy. After we did the VBAC preparation together, and everything was good. The second birth was so beautiful. It happened smoothly. I think it could happen because of the teamwork in that VBAC birth process.

If you have had a poor outcome of the mother or baby following a birth after caesarean, how did you cope with that and continue to support future women's birthing choices?

Never give judgemental statements that can hurt the mother. Offer support by convincing them that "she is not alone." Offering what things, we can do to help her matter. Because every mother needs different support.

What advice would you give clinicians reading the book on how to support women to have a better birth after a caesarean?

You must read this to know how and what the clinician should do to support the women to get a better birth after caesarean. Better is not always about the physical outcomes, but also mother's mental health and satisfaction in their birth process. Healing the previous birth by doing a better birth after caesarean. I think it's what really matters.

Vita Ratna Sari (Midwife) Reflection

Vita is a midwife coordinator of 5 years working at a general hospital in Surabaya, East Java.

Why do you think it is important to support women to have a better birth after caesarean?

Women have the right to reproductive health. These rights include the right to life, the right to equality, and freedom from all forms of discrimination, the right to obtain information and education, the right to marry or not marry, and form and plan a family, the right to decide whether to have children and when, the right to health services and protection. Birth by CS will indirectly have an impact on disrupting women's reproductive rights. Some of the impacts caused include disruption of the female reproductive system due to scars on the uterus. These wounds can later interfere with a woman's decision-making process about when to get pregnant or whether to have a limited number of children. Apart from that, Indonesia, which has ethnic and cultural diversity, still has a stigma that mothers who give birth by CS are not considered to be perfect mothers. This will lead to discrimination against women regarding their reproductive rights. So, women need to be supported to give birth better after CS surgery, to form and plan a healthy and prosperous family in the future. And she should be able to make decisions for herself.

What does a better birth after caesarean look like to you?

Normal delivery (VBAC) certainly has many benefits compared to subsequent delivery by CS. As midwives, we should be facilitators for women to provide an overview of the benefits and impacts of each birth, whether normal (VBAC) or CS. Next, it is hoped that women and their families will decide which one is best for them.

However, in practice in the field, it is not easy for me to provide such advocacy. I am a midwife who works in a government hospital in a city in Indonesia. At the hospital, we have specific guidelines created to support current government programs. We have special screening for complications in childbirth, including previous CS. All patients who have a history of BSC delivery are given a score and are required to deliver at a secondary health facility. Providers who provide obstetric services are mostly OB/GYN doctors. And most were given advice for giving birth by CS again. Apart from that, we who work in government agency health service facilities also have difficulties in providing comprehensive maternal pregnancy services with BSC related to health insurance system regulations.

For approximately 5 years I have worked in the delivery room. Some of the mothers who gave birth normally with BSC were mothers who came to the hospital with latent/active stage I or stage II conditions. So that labour will take place normally. Most mothers said they were satisfied with VBAC delivery. The mothers also stated that this was an extraordinary experience. How they, through their struggles, enjoyed the entire process of contractions in the first stage, the process in the second stage, and was able to carry out IMD directly (based on their experience, some births with CS did not carry out IMD). These mothers also said that they could interact with the baby and their families after the birth took place. This is different from previous deliveries. Some mothers felt sad about not being able to directly interact with their babies because of the influence of CS anaesthesia. So, it will also have an impact on the breastfeeding process. Another experience, the mother also said that she wanted to give birth normally again if the mother planned for the next pregnancy. Normal delivery has a faster recovery rate compared to CS and makes it easier for mothers to plan their next pregnancy.

How do you prepare women for a VBAC during pregnancy?

In Indonesia, the majority of pregnant women who have had a CS are referred to hospital during the second trimester of pregnancy. This is related to health insurance and the policies of each region. So, the care provided is less comprehensive to prepare for delivery with VBAC. This is because there are no specific national guidelines regarding IEC regarding birth options after CS or special screening that helps make it easier for health workers to facilitate mothers in choosing to give birth.

If a mother wants to give birth with a VBAC, we (midwives and OB/GYNs) at the secondary hospital help to screen first whether the mother is possible for a VBAC birth. This is related to the history of previous births, the cause of the choice of previous CS delivery, the age of the last child, comorbidities during pregnancy, etc. Next, we provide education regarding the benefits and risks of VBAC, and the actions and process of VBAC. General matters related to birth planning, such as preparation for childbirth and other support during pregnancy, which can later influence the VBAC process, such as nutritional status, complications of related diseases, such as preeclampsia, hypo/hyperthyroidism, etc. No less important is involving your husband or family in supporting the birthing process. This can help strengthen the mother's confidence in having a VBAC and support all the mother's needs before, during, and after the birth process.

How do you discuss with women who are planning a VBAC what a repeat caesarean may look like?

The first thing we do when women want and allow a VBAC is to provide education regarding the benefits and risks of VBAC, as well as the actions and process of VBAC. Education regarding the VBAC delivery process, including the risks of what happens if a VBAC delivery cannot occur and requires repeated CS surgery. In this way, the mother will prepare for all possible births. Apart from that, mothers are also expected to be able to make good decisions when this happens.

Is there a specific woman's better birth after caesarean that you remember? Why is that?

I'm not so sure about this. In certain cases, patients will be planned for an elective CS, such as pregnant women with CPD or with severe preeclampsia that cannot be regulated. This choice must inevitably be made by the mother with consideration for the welfare of the mother and her baby. Some of the experiences expressed by mothers were that mothers felt dissatisfied with their birth, such as not being able to perform IMD or feeling pain from the surgical scar. Apart from that, in Indonesia there is still a stigma that mothers who give birth via CS are not considered to be fully mothers. However, the mother is still grateful because she was able to give birth to a baby who was healthy and in good condition, without suffering from fatal complications.

If you have had a poor outcome of the mother or baby following a birth after caesarean, how did you cope with that and continue to support future women's birthing choices?

Each delivery option has its own risks, including CS. As midwives we try to minimize the risk of illness for mothers and babies. However, there are things that we cannot control along with the journey and process of action. We will support all decisions that are best for the mother, providing an overview of pregnancy planning until delivery that the mother can choose in the future. The initial counselling that we can do is to improve the mother's current condition. How to restore the health of the mother's reproductive organs first after the CS process. Education regarding nutrition, personal hygiene, contraception, and providing psychological support to mothers.

At our hospital, we have a policy to monitor the health condition of post-CS postpartum mothers with two visits to the hospital, namely in the first week and the second week after the mother returns from the hospital. This is a commitment to support the process of recovering the mother's condition. If the mother has special complications, such as preeclampsia, diabetes, etc., we will collaborate with midwives in the community to monitor the mother's health, as well as the condition of the baby.

What advice would you give clinicians reading the book on how to support women to have a better birth after caesarean?

Giving birth with VBAC is possible. The results of observations while working as a midwife show maternal satisfaction when experiencing a VBAC birth. Apart from that, a woman needs to be given support so that she is empowered to determine what is best for herself, especially choices regarding childbirth. I hope that this book can serve as a guide for clinicians in providing midwifery services. Clinicians are expected to have a broader perspective, especially regarding VBAC. Apart from that, I hope that through this book, clinicians can become good facilitators and advocates in fulfilling a woman's reproductive rights.

CHAPTER 11

Bringing it all Together

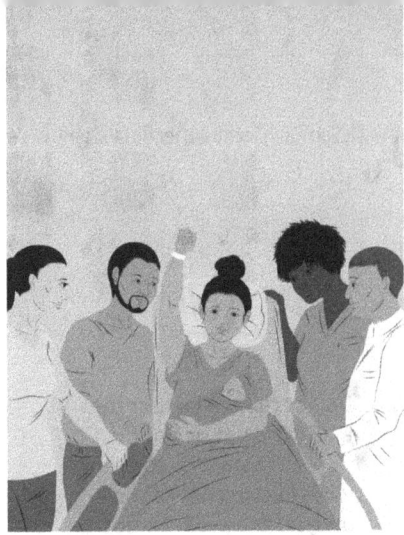

This concluding chapter will bring the previous chapters together by sharing experiences from women on why having a better birth after caesarean is important. It will discuss the ripple effect of having a positive, and often healing, birth on women lives.

Women's Advice to Clinicians on How to Support Better Birth after Caesarean

When I was writing this book, I reached out to Instagram to ask women what advice they would give clinicians regarding supporting their better birth after caesarean. I received many comments on the post, and many responses to the story. Below are some of the comments.

Look into a woman's previous birth information and be honest about the likelihood that it was interventions, and not her body "failing," that led to a caesarean. Tell her that no matter what happened last time, she has everything already within her to be able to have a vaginal birth.

Listen to want the woman wants or needs. Birth is about more than just the "mode of delivery." Awareness of the psychological impact of the previous birth which they may not be fully aware of until the next pregnancy.

Do not tell the birther that a VBAC is not an option. Do not tell them it is "too risky" whilst listing only cons and not the pros. Do not get consultants and other health care professionals to bully the birther into not having a VBAC.

Do not reel off stats in a way that makes them sound so much worse than they actually are. Do not only instil fear with regards to VBACs (you are very much made to feel like you are doing something incredibly irresponsible and reckless). Do not assume that the birther wants a repeat section. Do not keep trying to convince the birthing person that a VBAC is a "bad idea," and that they are risking their baby's life. Do not put the birthing person in the "high risk," and (my personal fave) "birthing outside of guidelines" box, because that is such a load of crap.

DO support, support, support. DO listen to the wants/wishes/desires of the birthing person. DO give them encouragement and belief. DO give them the pros as well as the cons.

DO speak positively about the option of a VBAC. And most of all, do not make it such a bloody fight to get there or that the birthing person feels their only option is to give in to the pressure of the system and/or another c-section. They should also read your book, Hazel, so that they actually have some sort of insight into VBAC, and how birthers really feel about this topic.

I could say so much more but I'll leave it at that!

Health care providers just need to understand where someone is coming from. Just stop, listen with openness and empathy and try and find a positive outcome for the person and their baby. Also, it's extremely condescending to act as if you're more invested in the baby's safety than the parents.

I believe the foundational attitude and assumption that you are capable of a successful VBAC needs to be the overarching theme from your health care providers so you feel empowered. Risk should absolutely be discussed, but within a context that isn't disproportionate and inflaming. Also, I think your health care provider should work with you to know how to advocate for whatever path you choose (e.g., monitoring choices, IV use, etc...) based on evidence and a woman's capacity to birth successfully after a caesarean.

Don't tell a woman who's had a CS that she won't be able to have a natural birth following. Encourage mothers to do research and provide accessible and positive stories, not just the fear- mongering ones. Let's mothers know they can actually say no, decline interventions at any time, and choose what interventions, if any, they would like for their VBAC, or simply decline all. Let VBAC patients know they can sign non-standard management plans that confirm they know the risks, but are happy to proceed.

Don't only talk about risks!! Share the successful incredible VBAC stories. The importance of picking your care provider, whether that be in hospital midwives or homebirth! Offer debriefing. Leave your bias aside. Get an understanding of background knowledge of your patient their fears, goals, culture, religion, etc ..., as these all effect birth. Also offer support to birth partners. Every birth and baby is different. Allow women to trust their bodies more! It's literally what they were created to do.

Acknowledgement of how the cascade of interventions and pressure very likely led to my c-section, even though I desperately tried to avoid them, but it was just too hard in the hospital system. Acknowledge and empower. More acknowledgement in general, that it is not ideal to lead women down the road to major abdominal surgery when it could be avoided, as it is not without its risks either. Both short-term and long-term.

Make sure you provide well rounded information, be mindful of terminology, and have a balanced conversation regarding supporting the woman's birth preference with absolute risk. (Had my 1st appointment, and already had them trying to push induction with not much response when I questioned why I'd do that when it increases likelihood of uterine rupture, which they're so concerned about, and telling me they'll have to see if I'm "allowed" to birth on MLU, despite me saying I don't want continuous monitoring. Not even 20 weeks yet—wasn't expecting this much of a fight on my hands.

Listen to the previous circum-stances and feelings around the caesarean, not just look at the medical notes. Discuss options and involve the mother in the planning. It's not just about getting a healthy baby at the end. It's about women feeling in control and part of the process. Using the BRAIN method of care too.

No being put on a time limit for dilation! And for the midwives and OBs to agree, as a team, on what's best for the patient. As I felt for me the midwives were working with me, but we ended up going with my OB's plan/strategy...ended up in another C-section ... even though mine and baby's vitals were normal. I just needed more time to "progress."

Also midwives (2 different midwives) internal dilation check was 4.5cm, and OBs was 2 to 3cm. How is that so different? Don't be so risk-averse that it impacts my birth!

If they could just understand the definition of coercion, that would be a great start. And that they should keep their opinions to themselves. Actual facts, if asked for.

Don't judge based on a prior birth. Each birth is so different. Anything saying failure to progress does not mean my body cannot progress the next time. Also, do not use negative verbiage like "trial of labour." Labour is labour. I believe in my body, and you should too!

Why wouldn't she be able to do it? It's very unlikely she won't be able to birth a baby she has grown herself. Understand statistics.

Not to call it a "trial" labour. Provide food during labour, if requested. Don't withhold for fear of eventual csection!

Have absolute trust that she CAN do it. Help her build that belief in herself. Find the actual

stats on risks so if other care providers try to frighten her, she already knows the truth. Tell her exactly what may come up in OB/hospital appts so she is prepared and doesn't feel blindsided.

I found "second-time" birthers were treated differently, with assumptions made about knowledge, preferences, etc ..., and fewer opportunities to discuss things as a result. People should be treated as first-time birthers unless they've requested otherwise. I hadn't had a VBAC or HBAC before, and so had lots of questions and new experiences.

Listen to women. Ask questions to understand their perspective and give personalised care. Don't just quote generic facts and statistics and hospital policies. After a difficult c-section, birthing women need to be supported, and have their power returned to them.

Just listen to us and also trust that we know our bodies best. Whatever we decide; if we feel supported and feel hard, we will be able to make more informed choices. Also, don't try and use stats to scare women into agreeing to any procedure they may not be comfortable with. Use good evidence-based advice tailored to their individual situation, and allow them the time and space to go away and be able to make informed decisions.

Supporting the decision of the mother if she decides to do a VBAC, without trying to pressure her into a repeat caesarean just because it is easy or it hasn't been the right amount of time between births.

Giving her the opportunity to decide what is right for her and supporting the way SHE wants to birth. Not everyone woman who has had an emergency caesarean wants another one because the first birth didn't work out.

Explore, listen, respect and advocate. Practice what you preach "Every pregnancy is different" :)

Don't fabricate or exaggerate the risks of VBAC to support your own personal opinion. Also don't play down the risks of caesarean birth (especially after two or more previous caesareans). Prioritise true informed consent over fear. Give women the true, transparent statistics, and then support them in whatever their informed decision may be.

I'd hope that the information being given to me was supported by up-to-date, quality, evidence-based research and given without judgement or scare tactics. When you're pregnant, you will do whatever you can to protect your baby. We put a lot of trust in clinicians in our care team. Your individual needs can be easily dismissed due to the perceived risk of VBAC births.

Believing that VBAC is possible as a baseline, not an exception! Tell me that I can do it, and the steps that I can take to increase my chances. Don't be so risk-averse that it impacts my birth.

Undertake support training to better understand what a woman having a VBAC needs—actually look at the individual in front of you and understand their needs ... not just a medical point of view, and especially if a repeat needs to occur, actually think of the emotional impact of this and ways to provide additional support. - Move some mountains to let another support person into surgery, ensure skin to skin is happening, DCC, and is there an opportunity for maternal assistance.

Give actual numbers rather than saying "risk doubles, etc."

Don't say if it was me, "I would do this."

If there isn't any evidence for the choice being made, state that.

Ensure they have as much info as possible to optimise their next birth experience (whatever this might be, - e.g., if planning a VBAC), inform them how being in their own environment with birth support who value physiology and hormones.

If choosing repeat caesarean, inform them on the positive benefits of skin to skin, delayed cord clamping, maternal- assisted caesarean, etc... Good luck..

Can they also understand CTG use and VBACs better too.

Crucial conversations about products available in the community setting, that HCPs don't recommend. Why? Because of silly rules like endorsement policies.

As an experienced VBAC midwife, I feel a thorough non-judgmental debriefing about the previous C/S is important. Especially for the woman and partner to express how they felt. A quick rundown on the so called "risks" of VBAC without all the negative carry on, and then pop them in a box and put a lid on it. A discussion about physiological birth, especially oxytocin and birth room environment, is very important. A well planned VBAC can be quickly undermined by idiot doctors or midwives who aren't on the same page, and come into the birth room exuding anxiety!

Listen, and ask the woman why she wants a certain birth; what it means to her, and why it's important. Ask her how

many children she wants. Be clear, open, and transparent in a compassionate way. Be supportive, understand, and actually want to help the woman achieve the birth she wants. Learn all you can to support the woman have that birth. If you don't have confidence in her choice, research why you don't have confidence. Is it bias? Lack of understanding? Clash of birth values? If you can't support a woman in that capacity, match her with someone who will give her the best chance.

Asking just that, how best can I support you?

I Felt Like Superwoman!

In my first research project, the HBAC study, I interviewed women who had a VBAC at home. One of the questions I asked, which often came after they had shared their long journeys from pain to power, was *"how did you feel after having your VBAC at home?"* I watched the women draw in a big breath, sit a little taller, smile, and say the most empowering things. I loved asking that question, and when I listened back to the interviews, these comments got me teary.

When I would present at conferences on the research, I would play a soundbite of the responses, and the audience would have such a big reaction. There would be tears, smiles, and nods of recognition. Once I started presenting on my PhD, I forgot about the soundbite. But at a recent conference where I was invited to speak, a wonderful midwife reminded me of it and said how she loved hearing it back in the day! I found it, popped it in the presentation, and loved seeing the reaction in the audience.

I have the words below, it's not the same as hearing the pride and joy in their voices. You will need to imagine that. The sentiments are there, though. If you have got to the end of this book (or love reading the end first), and you are still not sure why VBAC is important, please absorb the power and joy in their responses.

Hazel:
How did you feel after having a VBAC at home?

Woman 1:
Euphoric. Absolutely euphoric. It was amazing. It really was.

Woman 2:
It was just overwhelming. It was just the most magical experience. Absolutely awesome. It was everything that I wanted it to be.

Woman 3:
Ecstatic. Powerful. I don't think I came back down to Earth for about 2 weeks.

Woman 4:
Awesome. It was the most amazing experience. Amazing. Amazing. No drugs, just wonderful.

Woman 5:
Yeah. It just felt very normal, I suppose. That's the best way I could describe it.

Woman 6:
Wow. Yeah, it was great, and it was very positive, and it was relaxed. And yeah, it was a really healing experience, which I suppose is what most people would've felt really normal and good. Yeah.

Woman 7:
Just blown away. It was mind-blowing. Best experience of my life, and it wasn't because it was a VBAC, it was because it was just giving birth.

Woman 8:
I felt like I needed to run around with a big fat, "I told you so." To my GP, to everybody. I felt like finally I could relate to a lot of the mothers I know who have given birth vaginally. And actually, I felt I had one up on them, because they did it in hospital under ... I felt like I had one up on them.

Woman 9:
I felt like Superwoman! It was wonderful. It was wonderful.

Woman 10:
Fantastic. This is the best thing that's ever happened, and I want everyone in the whole world to know how fantastic this is. And the high was just so high. It stayed as one of the best moments of my life still. And that was 4 and a half years ago. I would not ever forget how amazed I was to have actually done it.

Woman 11:
You feel so happy and complete. And I got to enter into this not club, but I feel like this is what I was meant to do as a woman. Not just to have the baby at the end of it, but actually to give birth to my own child.

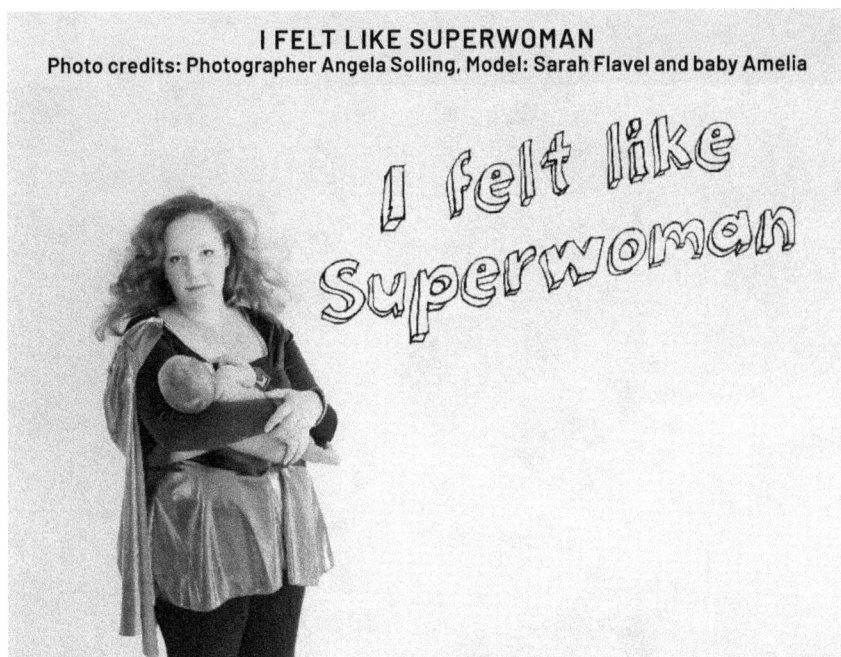

I FELT LIKE SUPERWOMAN
Photo credits: Photographer Angela Solling, Model: Sarah Flavel and baby Amelia

Summary

This book has been a joy to write. It had been a couple of years since I wrote my first book, and in that time, I have been a busy academic with a family of teenagers. Time to sit and write, without endless meetings and emails, was very hard to find! Carving out time to take a deep dive back into the research on birth after caesarean was a wonderful experience.

I hope you have found the book helpful. It is meant to be a combination of evidence, reflection points, clinicians' stories, and women's advice alongside my personal thoughts, stories, and suggestions. I'm hoping that combination worked for you! I hope that you share this with other colleagues and clinicians across disciplines so that in the future all women can be provided with respectful maternity care.

Please stay in touch, I would love to hear how you found the book. You can find me on Instagram at @hazelkeedle.

Now go and support women to have their best birth after caesarean! You've got this!

References

Aboshama, R. A., Taha, O. T., Abdel Halim, H. W., Elrehim, E. I. A., Kamal, S. H. M., Elsherbiny, A. M., Magdy, H. A., Albayadi, E., Elsaid, R. E., Abdelghany, A. M., Anan, M. A., & Abdelfattah, L. E. (2023). Prevalence and risk factor of postoperative adhesions following repeated cesarean section: A prospective cohort study. *International Journal of Gynecology & Obstetrics*, *161*(1), 234-240. https://doi.org/10.1002/ijgo.14498

ACOG. (2010). *Practice bulletin: Vaginal birth after previous cesarean delivery* (Obstetrics & Gynecology, Issue.

ACOG. (2017). *Practice bulletin No. 184: Vaginal birth after cesarean delivery*. I. Wolters Kluwer Health. https://www.acog.org/Womens-Health/Vaginal-Birth-After-Cesarean-VBAC

ACOG. (2019). *Vaginal birth after cesarean delivery* (1873-233X). (Obstetrics and gynecology (Online), Issue.

Adams, C., & Curtin-Bowen, M. (2021). Countervailing powers in the labor room: The doula-doctor relationship in the United States. *Social Science & Medicine*, *285*, 114296. https://doi.org/10.1016/j.socscimed.2021.114296

Adjei, N. N., McMillan, C., Hosier, H., Partridge, C., Adeyemo, O. O., & Illuzzi, J. (2023). Assessing the predictive accuracy of the new vaginal birth after cesarean delivery calculator. *American Journal of Obstetrics & Gynecology, Maternal-Fetal Medicine (MFM)*, *5*(6), 100960. https://doi.org/10.1016/j.ajogmf.2023.100960

Ahlers-Schmidt, C. R., Woods, N. K., Bradshaw, D., Rempel, A., Engel, M., & Benton, M. (2018). Maternal knowledge, attitudes, and practices concerning interpregnancy interval. *Kansas Journal of Medicine*, *11*(4), 86.

AIHW. (2024). *Australia's mothers and babies 2022*. https://www.aihw.gov.au/reports-data/population-groups/mothers-babies/overview

Akhavan, S., & Edge, D. (2012). Foreign-born women's experiences of community-based doulas in Sweden—A qualitative study. *Health Care for Women International*, *33*(9), 833-848. https://doi.org/10.1080/07399332.2011.646107

Alfirevic, Z., Gyte, G. M. L., Cuthbert, A., & Devane, D. (2017). Continuous cardiotocography (CTG) as a form of electronic fetal monitoring (EFM) for fetal assessment during labour. *Cochrane Database of Systematic Reviews*(2). https://doi.org/10.1002/14651858.CD006066.pub3 Andersen, M. M., Thisted, D. L. A., Amer-Wåhlin, I., & Krebs, L. (2016). Can Intrapartum cardiotocography predict uterine rupture among women with prior caesarean delivery?: A population based case-control study. *PLoS One*, *11*(2), e0146347. https://doi.org/10.1371/journal.pone.0146347

Angolile, C. M., Max, B. L., Mushemba, J., & Mashauri, H. L. (2023). Global increased cesarean section rates and public health implications: A call to action. *Health Science Reports*, *6*(5). https://doi.org/10.1002/hsr2.1274

Antoine, C., & Young, B. K. (2021). Cesarean section one hundred years 1920–2020: The good, the bad and the ugly. *Journal of Perinatal Medicine*, *49*(1), 5-16. https://doi.

org/10.1515/jpm-2020-0305

Aseffa, F., Mehari, L., Gure, F., & Wylie, L. (2024). Racism in Ontario midwifery: Indigenous, black and racialized midwives and midwifery students unsilenced. *Canadian Journal of Midwifery Research and Practice, 20*(2), 10-22. https://doi.org/10.22374/cjmrp.v20i2.44

Ayerle, G. M., Mattern, E., Striebich, S., Oganowski, T., Ocker, R., Haastert, B., Schafers, R., & Seliger, G. (2023). Effect of alternatively designed hospital birthing rooms on the rate of vaginal births: Multicentre randomised controlled trial Be-Up. *Women & Birth, 36*(5), 429-438. https://doi.org/10.1016/j.wombi.2023.02.009

Bannister, L., Hammond, A., Dahlen, H., Keedle, H. (2025) A content analysis of women's experiences of debriefing following childbirth: The birth experience study (BESt). *Midwifery, 146.* https://doi.org/10.1016/j.midw.2025.104421

Barger, M. K., Dunn, J. T., Bearman, S., Delain, M., & Gates, E. (2013). A survey of access to trial of labor in California hospitals in 2012. *BMC Pregnancy Childbirth, 13*(1), 83. https://doi.org/10.1186/1471-2393-13-83

Bayrampour, H., Lisonkova, S., Tamana, S., Wines, J., Vedam, S., & Janssen, P. (2021). Perinatal outcomes of planned home birth after cesarean and planned hospital vaginal birth after cesarean at term gestation in British Columbia, Canada: A retrospective population based cohort study. *Birth.* https://doi.org/10.1111/birt.12539

Bayri Bingol, F., Demirgoz Bal, M., Aygun, M., & Bilgic, E. (2021). Secondary traumatic stress among midwifery students. *Perspectives in Psychiatric Care, 57*(3), 1195-1201. https://doi.org/10.1111/ppc.12674

Beck, C. T. (2004). Birth trauma: In the eye of the beholder. *Nursing Research, 53*(1), 28-35.

Beckmann, L., Barger, M., Dorin, L., Metzing, S., & Hellmers, C. (2014). Vaginal Birth after cesarean in German out-of-hospital settings: Maternal and neonatal outcomes of women with their second child. *Birth.* https://doi.org/10.1111/birt.12130

Bell, C. H., Dahlen, H. G., & Davis, D. (2023). Finding a way forward for the birth plan and maternal decision making: A discussion paper. *Midwifery, 126,* 103806. https://doi.org/10.1016/j.midw.2023.103806

Bell, C. H., Muggleton, S., & Davis, D. L. (2022). Birth plans: A systematic, integrative review into their purpose, process, and impact. *Midwifery, 111,* 103388. https://doi.org/10.1016/j.midw.2022.103388

Blake, J. A., Gardner, M., Najman, J., & Scott, J. G. (2021). The association of birth by caesarean section and cognitive outcomes in offspring: a systematic review. *Social Psychiatry and Psychiatric Epidemiology, 56*(4), 533-545. https://doi.org/10.1007/s00127-020-02008-2

Blazkova, B., Pastorkova, A., Solansky, I., Veleminsky, M., Rossnerova, A., Honkova, K., Rossner, P., & Sram, R. J. (2020). The impact of cesarean and vaginal delivery on results of psychological cognitive test in 5-year-old children. *Medicina, 56*(10), 554.

Bohren, M. A., Hofmeyr, G. J., Sakala, C., Fukuzawa, R. K., & Cuthbert, A. (2017). Continuous support for women during childbirth. *Cochrane Database of Systematic reviews*, *2017*(8). https://doi.org/10.1002/14651858.cd003766.pub6

Boley, J. (1935). The history of caesarean section. *Canadian Medical Association Journal*, *32*(5), 557.

Brown, A., Nielsen, J. D. J., Russo, K., Ayers, S., & Webb, R. (2022). The Journey towards resilience following a traumatic birth: A grounded theory. *Midwifery*, *104*, 103204. https://doi.org/10.1016/j.midw.2021.103204

Brown, K., Langston Cox, A., & Unger, H. W. (2021). A better start to life: Risk factors for, and prevention of, preterm birth in Australian First Nations women – A narrative review. *International Journal of Gynecology & Obstetrics*, *155*(2), 260-267. https://doi.org/10.1002/ijgo.13907

Buran, G., & Aksu, H. (2022). Effect of hypnobirthing training on fear, pain, satisfaction related to birth, and birth outcomes: A randomized-controlled trial. *Clinical Nursing Research*, *31*(5), 918-930. https://doi.org/10.1177/10547738211073394

Byrskog, U., Small, R., & Schytt, E. (2020). Community-based bilingual doulas for migrant women in labour and birth – Findings from a Swedish register-based cohort study. *BMC Pregnancy Childbirth*, *20*(1). https://doi.org/10.1186/s12884-020-03412-x

Carlsson, T., & Ulfsdottir, H. (2020). Waterbirth in low risk pregnancy: An exploration of women's experiences. *Journal of Advanced Nursing*, *76*(5), 1221-1231. https://doi.org/10.1111/jan.14336

Chamagne, M., Richard, M. B., Vallee, A., Tahiri, J., Renevier, B., Dahlhoff, S., Garcia, D., Vivanti, A., & Ayoubi, J. M. (2023). Trial of labour versus elective caesarean delivery for estimated large for gestational age foetuses after prior caesarean delivery: A multicenter retrospective study. *BMC Pregnancy Childbirth*, *23*(1). https://doi.org/10.1186/s12884-023-05688-1

Chang, Y. H. (2020). Uterine rupture over 11 years: A retrospective descriptive study. *Australian and New Zealand Journal of Obstetrics and Gynaecology*, *60*(5), 709-713. https://doi.org/10.1111/ajo.13133

Cheyney, M., Bovbjerg, M., Everson, C., Gordon, W., Hannibal, D., & Vedam, S. (2014). Outcomes of care for 16,924 planned home births in the United States: The Midwives Alliance of North America Statistics Project, 2004 to 2009. *Journal of Midwifery & Women's Health*, *59*(1), 17-27. https://doi.org/10.1111/jmwh.12172

Christoph, P., Aebi, J., Sutter, L., Schmitt, K.-U., Surbek, D., & Oelhafen, S. (2023). The extended gentle caesarean section protocol—expanding the scope and adding value for the family: A cross-sectional study. *Archives of Gynecology and Obstetrics*, *307*(5), 1481-1488. https://doi.org/10.1007/s00404-023-06913-0

Chu, J., Keedle, H., Sutcliffe, K., Blumenthal, N., & Levett, K. (2024). The outcomes for women planning a VBAC at a private hospital in Australia. *Birth*. https://doi.org/10.1111/birt.12811

Clews, C., Church, S., & Ekberg, M. (2019). Women and waterbirth: A systematic meta-synthesis of qualitative studies. *Women and Birth*. https://doi.org/10.1016/j.wombi.2019.11.007

Coddington, R., Scarf, V., & Fox, D. (2023). Australian women's experiences of wearing a non-invasive fetal electrocardiography (NIFECG) device during labour. *Women and Birth, 36*(6), 546-551. https://doi.org/https://doi.org/10.1016/j.wombi.2023.03.005

Cohen, N. W., & Estner, L. J. (1983). *Silent knife: Cesarean prevention and vaginal birth after cesarean (VBAC)*. Bergin & Garvey Publishers.

Cooper, M., McCutcheon, H., & Warland, J. (2021). 'They follow the wants and needs of an institution': Midwives' views of water immersion. *Women & Birth, 34*(2), e178-e187. https://doi.org/10.1016/j.wombi.2020.02.019

Cooper, M., & Warland, J. (2019). What are the benefits? Are they concerned? Women's experiences of water immersion for labor and birth. *Midwifery, 79*, 102541. https://doi.org/10.1016/j.midw.2019.102541

Cragin, E., B. (1916). Conservatism in Obstetrics. *New York Medical Journal, 104*, 1-3. https://archive.org/details/newyorkmedicaljo1041unse/page/n7/mode/2up?view=theater&q=cragin

Cunningham, F. G., Bangdiwala, S. I., Brown, S. S., Dean, T. M., Frederiksen, M., Rowland, C. H., King, T., Spencer, E. L., McCullough, L. B., & Nicholson, W. (2010). NIH consensus development conference draft statement on vaginal birth after cesarean: New insights. *NIH Consensus and State-of-the-Science Statements, 27*(3), 1-42. https://uncch.pure.elsevier.com/en/publications/nih-consensus-development-conference-draft-statement-on-vaginal-b

Cunningham, J., Calestani, D. M., & Coxon, D. K. (2024). How experiences of weight stigma impact higher-weight women during their maternity care: A meta-ethnography. *Midwifery, 141*, 104242. https://doi.org/10.1016/j.midw.2024.104242

Darwin, Z., Green, J., McLeish, J., Willmot, H., & Spiby, H. (2017). Evaluation of trained volunteer doula services for disadvantaged women in five areas in England: women's experiences. *Health, Social Care, & Community, 25*(2), 466-477. https://doi.org/10.1111/hsc.12331

Davis-Floyd, R. (1993). The technocratic model of birth. *Childbirth: Changing ideas and practices in britain and america 1600 to the present.* In S.T. Hollis, L. Pershing, and M.J. Young (Eds.) *Feminist theory in the study of folklore* (pp. 247-276). U. of Illinois Press. Davis, D.-A. (2019). Obstetric racism: The racial politics of pregnancy, labor, and birthing. *Medical Anthropology, 38*(7), 560-573. https://doi.org/10.1080/01459740.2018.1549389

Davis, D.-A. (2020). Reproducing while Black: the crisis of Black maternal health, obstetric racism and assisted reproductive technology. *Reproductive Biomedicine & Society Online, 11*, 56-64. https://doi.org/https://doi.org/10.1016/j.rbms.2020.10.001

Desseauve, D., Bonifazi-Grenouilleau, M., Fritel, X., Lathélize, J., Sarreau, M., & Pierre, F. (2016). Fetal heart rate abnormalities associated with uterine rupture: a case–control study: A new time-lapse approach using a standardized classification. *European Journal of Obstetrics & Gynecology and Reproductive Biology, 197*, 16-21. https://doi.org/https://doi.org/10.1016/j.ejogrb.2015.10.019

Dixon, L., Daellenbach, S., Anderson, J., Neely, E., Nisa-Waller, A., & Lockwood, S.

(2023). Building positive respectful midwifery relationships: An analysis of women's experiences of continuity of midwifery care in Aotearoa New Zealand. *Women & Birth, 36*(6), e669-e675. https://doi.org/10.1016/j.wombi.2023.06.008

Djatmika, C., Lusher, J., Williamson, H., & Harcourt, D. (2024). 'Plan Z and then off the edge of a cliff': An interpretative phenomenological analysis of mothers' experience of living with a slow-to-heal caesarean wound. *Midwifery, 137,* 104104. https://doi.org/10.1016/j.midw.2024.104104

Dmowska, A., Fielding-Singh, P., Halpern, J., & Prata, N. (2023). The intersection of traumatic childbirth and obstetric racism: A qualitative study. *Birth.* https://doi.org/10.1111/birt.12774

Dong, H., Song, J., Jia, Y., Cui, H., & Chen, X. (2024). A comprehensive study on the risk factors and pathogen analysis of postoperative wound infections following caesarean section procedures. *International Wound Journal, 21*(1). https://doi.org/10.1111/iwj.14609

Dunning, T., Martin, H., & McGrath, Y. (2019). Vaginal birth after caesarean: How NICE guidelines can inform midwifery practice. *British Journal of Midwifery, 27*(11), 689-693. https://doi.org/10.12968/bjom.2019.27.11.689

Edqvist, M., Dahlen, H. G., Haggsgard, C., Tern, H., Angeby, K., Teleman, P., Ajne, G., & Rubertsson, C. (2022). The effect of two midwives during the second stage of labour to reduce severe perineal trauma (Oneplus): A multicentre, randomised controlled trial in Sweden. *Lancet, 399*(10331), 1242-1253. https://doi.org/10.1016/S0140-6736(22)00188-X

Elphinstone, D. N. (2023). Maternal-assisted caesareans. *The Practising Midwife Australia, 2*(1), 8-11. https://doi.org/10.55975/emsp4141

Elvander, C., Ahlberg, M., Edqvist, M., & Stephansson, O. (2019). Severe perineal trauma among women undergoing vaginal birth after cesarean delivery: A population-based cohort study. *Birth, 46*(2), 379-386. https://doi.org/10.1111/birt.12402

Elvander, C., Ahlberg, M., Thies-Lagergren, L., Cnattingius, S., & Stephansson, O. (2015). Birth position and obstetric anal sphincter injury: AW population-based study of 113,000 spontaneous births. *BMC Pregnancy & Childbirth, 15*(1). https://doi.org/10.1186/s12884-015-0689-7

Ertan, D., Hingray, C., Burlacu, E., Sterlé, A., & El-Hage, W. (2021). Post-traumatic stress disorder following childbirth. *BMC Psychiatry, 21*(1). https://doi.org/10.1186/s12888-021-03158-6

Euro-Peristat Project. (2022). *European Perinatal Health Report: Core indicators of the health and care of pregnant women and babies in Europe from 2015 to 2019.* https://www.europeristat.com/

Euro-Peristat Project. (2018). *European perinatal health report: core indicators of the health and care of pregnant women and babies in Europe in 2015.* https://www.europeristat.com/images/EPHR2015_web_hyperlinked_Euro-Peristat.pdf

Facchetti, G., Teo, Z., Sharma, M., & Budden, A. (2024). Continuity obstetric care demonstrates greater vaginal birth after caesarean success. *Australian and New Zealand Journal of Obstetrics and Gynaecology, 64*(3), 264-268. https://doi.org/10.1111/ajo.13790

Fagerberg, M. C., Marsal, K., & Kallen, K. (2015). Predicting the chance of vaginal delivery after one cesarean section: validation and elaboration of a published prediction model. *European Journal of Obstetrics,Gynecology, & Reproductive Biology*, *188*, 88-94. https://doi.org/10.1016/j.ejogrb.2015.02.031

Fair, C. D., Crawford, A., Houpt, B., & Latham, V. (2020). "After having a waterbirth, I feel like it's the only way people should deliver babies": The decision making process of women who plan a waterbirth. *Midwifery*, *82*, 102622. https://doi.org/10.1016/j.midw.2019.102622

Farid Mojtahedi, M., Sepidarkish, M., Almukhtar, M., Eslami, Y., Mohammadianamiri, F., Behzad Moghadam, K., Rouholamin, S., Razavi, M., Jafari Tadi, M., Fazlollahpour-Naghibi, A., Rostami, Z., Rostami, A., & Rezaeinejad, M. (2023). Global incidence of surgical site infections following caesarean section: A systematic review and meta-analysis. *Journal of Hospital Infections*, *139*, 82-92. https://doi.org/10.1016/j.jhin.2023.05.019

Felstead, K. T. (2020). *Young mothers: Discursive constructions of their lives and identities* Federation University Australia]. Victoria.

Ferguson, B., Baldwin, A., Henderson, A., & Harvey, C. (2022). The grounded theory of Coalescence of Perceptions, Practice and Power: An understanding of governance in midwifery practice. *Journal of Nursing Management*, *30*(8), 4587-4594. https://doi.org/10.1111/jonm.13892

Fitzpatrick, K. E., Kurinczuk, J. J., Bhattacharya, S., & Quigley, M. A. (2019). Planned mode of delivery after previous cesarean section and short-term maternal and perinatal outcomes: A population-based record linkage cohort study in Scotland. *PLoS Med*, *16*(9), e1002913. https://doi.org/10.1371/journal.pmed.1002913

Foureur, M., Ryan, C.L., Nicholl, M., Homer, C. (2010). Inconsistent evidence: Analysis of six national guidelines for Vaginal Birth After Cesarean Section. *Birth*, *37*(1), 3-8.

Fox, D., Coddington, R., Levett, K. M., Scarf, V., Sutcliffe, K. L., & Newnham, E. (2024). Tending to the machine: The impact of intrapartum fetal surveillance on women in Australia. *PLoS One*, *19*(5), e0303072. https://doi.org/10.1371/journal.pone.0303072

Fox, D., Coddington, R., & Scarf, V. (2021). Wanting to be 'with woman', not with machine: Midwives' experiences of caring for women being continuously monitored in labour. *Women & Birth*. https://doi.org/10.1016/j.wombi.2021.09.002

Fox, D., Coddington, R., Scarf, V., Bisits, A., Lainchbury, A., Woodworth, R., Maude, R., Foureur, M., & Sandall, J. (2021). Harnessing technology to enable all women mobility in labour and birth: Feasibility of implementing beltless non-invasive fetal ECG applying the NASSS framework. *Pilot and Feasibility Studies*, *7*(1). https://doi.org/10.1186/s40814-021-00953-6

Fox, N. S. (2020). Pregnancy Outcomes in Patients With Prior Uterine Rupture or Dehiscence: A 5-Year Update. *Obstetrics & Gynecology*, *135*(1), 211-212. https://doi.org/10.1097/AOG.0000000000003622

Fox, N. S., Gerber, R. S., Mourad, M., Saltzman, D. H., Klauser, C. K., Gupta, S., &

Rebarber, A. (2014). Pregnancy outcomes in patients with prior uterine rupture or dehiscence. *Obstetrics & Gynecology, 123*(4), 785-789. https://doi.org/10.1097/AOG.0000000000000181

Friedman, E. A., & Cohen, W. R. (2023). Dysfunctional labor and delivery: adverse effects on offspring. *American Journal of Obstetrics and Gynecology, 228*(5), S1104-S1109. https://doi.org/10.1016/j.ajog.2022.10.011

Goldkuhl, L., Dellenborg, L., Berg, M., Wijk, H., & Nilsson, C. (2022). The influence and meaning of the birth environment for nulliparous women at a hospital-based labour ward in Sweden: An ethnographic study. *Women & Birth, 35*(4), e337-e347. https://doi.org/10.1016/j.wombi.2021.07.005

Gregory, K. D., Fridman, M., & Korst, L. (2010). Trends and patterns of vaginal birth after cesarean availability in the United States. *Seminars in Perinatology, 34*(4), 237-243. https://doi.org/10.1053/j.semperi.2010.03.002

Grenvik, J. M., Coleman, L. A., & Berghella, V. (2023). Birthing balls to decrease labor pain and peanut balls to decrease length of labor: What is the evidence? *American Journal of Obstetrics and Gynecology, 228*(5), S1270-S1273. https://doi.org/10.1016/j.ajog.2023.02.014

Grenvik, J. M., Rosenthal, E., Wey, S., Saccone, G., De Vivo, V., De Prisco Lcp, A., Delgado Garcia, B. E., & Berghella, V. (2022). Birthing ball for reducing labor pain: A systematic review and meta-analysis of randomized controlled trials. *Journal of Maternal Fetal & Neonatal Medicine, 35*(25), 5184-5193. https://doi.org/10.1080/14767058.2021.1875439

Grobman, L. Y., Landon, M., Spong, C., Leveno, K., Rouse, D., Varner, M., Moawad, A., Caritis, S., Harper, M., Wapner, R., Sorokin, Y., Miodovnik, M., Carpenter, M., O'Sullivan, M., Sibai, B., Langer, O., Thorp, J., & Ramin, S., (2007). Development of a nomogram for prediction of Vaginal Birth After Cesarean Delivery. *Obstetrics and Gynecology, 109*(4), 806-812.

Grobman, W. A., Sandoval, G., Rice, M. M., Bailit, J. L., Chauhan, S. P., Costantine, M. M., Gyamfi-Bannerman, C., Metz, T. D., Parry, S., Rouse, D. J., Saade, G. R., Simhan, H. N., Thorp, J. M., Tita, A. T. N., Longo, M., & Landon, M. B. (2021). Prediction of vaginal birth after cesarean delivery in term gestations: A calculator without race and ethnicity. *American Journal of Obstetrics and Gynecology.* https://doi.org/10.1016/j.ajog.2021.05.021

Guiliano, M., Closset, E., Therby, D., LeGoueff, F., Deruelle, P., & Subtil, D. (2014). Signs, symptoms and complications of complete and partial uterine ruptures during pregnancy and delivery. *European Journal of Obstetrics, Gynecology, & Reproductive Biology, 179C*, 130-134. https://doi.org/10.1016/j.ejogrb.2014.05.004

Habteyes, A. T., Mekuria, M. D., Negeri, H. A., Kassa, R. T., Deribe, L. K., & Sendo, E. G. (2024). Prevalence and associated factors of caesarean section among mothers who gave birth across Eastern Africa countries: Systematic review and meta-analysis study. *Heliyon, 10*(12), e32511. https://doi.org/10.1016/j.heliyon.2024.e32511

Hardeman, R. R., & Kozhimannil, K. B. (2016). Motivations for entering the doula profession: Perspectives from women of color. *Journal of Midwifery & Women's*

Health, 61(6), 773-780. https://doi.org/10.1111/jmwh.12497

Heelan Fancher, L., Shi, L., Zhang, Y., Cai, Y., Nawai, A., & Leveille, S. (2019). Impact of continuous electronic fetal monitoring on birth outcomes in low risk pregnancies. *Birth, 46*(2), 311-317. https://doi.org/10.1111/birt.12422

Hoang, D. M., Levy, E. I., & Vandenplas, Y. (2021). The impact of caesarean section on the infant gut microbiome. *Acta Paediatrica, 110*(1), 60-67. https://doi.org/10.1111/apa.15501

Hochler, H., Tevet, A., Barg, M., Suissa-Cohen, Y., Lipschuetz, M., Yagel, S., Aviram, A., Mei-Dan, E., Melamed, N., Barrett, J. F. R., Fox, N. S., & Walfisch, A. (2022). Trial of labor of vertex-nonvertex twins following a previous cesarean delivery. *American Journal of Obstetrics & Gynecology, Maternal Fetal Medicine (MFM), 4*(4), 100640. https://doi.org/10.1016/j.ajogmf.2022.100640

Hodgson, Z. G., Comfort, L. R., & Albert, A. A. Y. (2020). Water birth and perinatal outcomes in British Columbia: A retrospective cohort study. *Journal of Obstetrics & Gynaecology Canada, 42*(2), 150-155. https://doi.org/10.1016/j.jogc.2019.07.007

Homer, C. S. E., Davis, D. L., Mollart, L., Turkmani, S., Smith, R. M., Bullard, M., Leiser, B., & Foureur, M. (2021). Midwifery continuity of care and vaginal birth after caesarean section: A randomised controlled trial. *Women and Birth.* https://doi.org/10.1016/j.wombi.2021.05.010

Horgan, R., Hossain, S., Fulginiti, A., Patras, A., Massaro, R., Abuhamad, A. Z., Kawakita, T., & Graebe, R. (2022). Trial of labor after two cesarean sections: A retrospective case–control study. *Journal of Obstetrics and Gynaecology Research, 48*(10), 2528-2533. https://doi.org/10.1111/jog.15351

Hsu, I., Hsu, L., Dorjee, S., & Hsu, C.-C. (2022). Bacterial colonization at caesarean section defects in women of secondary infertility: an observational study. *BMC Pregnancy & Childbirth, 22*(1). https://doi.org/10.1186/s12884-022-04471-y

Iida, M., Horiuchi, S., & Nagamori, K. (2014). A comparison of midwife-led care versus obstetrician-led care for low-risk women in Japan. *Women and Birth, 27*(3), 202-207. https://doi.org/https://doi.org/10.1016/j.wombi.2014.05.001 (Women and Birth)

International Confederation of Midwives. (2024). *Obstetric violence and mistreatment and violence against women in reproductive health services.* https://internationalmidwives.org/resources/obstetric-violence-and-mistreatment-and-violence-against-women-in-reproductive-health-services/

James, E. (2020). *A hermeneutic phenomenological study into the midwife-woman relationship.* Auckland University of Technology]. Auckland.

Jauniaux, E., Jurkovic, D., Hussein, A. M., & Burton, G. J. (2022). New insights into the etiopathology of placenta accreta spectrum. *American Journal of Obstetrics & Gynecology, 227*(3), 384-391. https://doi.org/10.1016/j.ajog.2022.02.038

Jordan, B. (1997). Authoritative Knowledge and Its Construction. In R. Davis-Floyd & C. Sargent (Eds.), *Childbirth and authoritative knowledge: Cross-cultural perspectives.* University of California Press.

Kang, E., Stowe, N. E., Burton, K., & Ritchwood, T. D. (2024). Characterizing the utilization of doula support services among birthing people of color in the United States: A scoping review. *BMC Public Health*, *24*(1). https://doi.org/10.1186/s12889-024-19093-6

Keedle, Schmied, V., Burns, E., & Dahlen, H. (2018a). The design, development, and evaluation of a qualitative data collection application for pregnant women. *Journal of Nursing Scholarship*, *50*(1), 47-55. https://doi.org/10.1111/jnu.12344

Keedle, Schmied, V., Burns, E., & Dahlen, H. (2018b). The journey from pain to power: A meta-ethnography on women's experiences of vaginal birth after caesarean. *Women and Birth*, *31*(1), 69-79. https://doi.org/https://doi.org/10.1016/j.wombi.2017.06.008

Keedle, Schmied, V., Burns, E., & Dahlen, H. G. (2015). Women's reasons for, and experiences of, choosing a homebirth following a caesarean section. *BMC Pregnancy & Childbirth*, *15*(1), 206. https://doi.org/10.1186/s12884-015-0639-4

Keedle, H. (2022). *Birth after caesarean: Your journey to a better birth.* Praeclarus Press.

Keedle, H., & Dahlen, H. (2023). *Submission to the NSW Inquiry into Birth Trauma* [Report]. Western Sydney University.

Keedle, H., Keedle, W., & Dahlen, H. G. (2024). Dehumanized, violated, and powerless: An Australian survey of women's experiences of obstetric violence in the past 5 years. *Violence Against Women*, *30*(9), 2320-2344. https://doi.org/10.1177/10778012221140138

Keedle, H., Lockwood, R., Keedle, W., Susic, D., & Dahlen, H. (2023). What women want if they were to have another baby: The Australian Birth Experience Study (BESt) cross-sectional national survey. *BMJ Open*. https://doi.org/10.1136/bmjopen-2023-071582

Keedle, H., Peters, L., Schmied, V., Burns, E., Keedle, W., & Dahlen, H. (2020a). Women's experiences of planning a vaginal birth after caesarean in different models of maternity care in Australia. *BMC Pregnancy & Childbirth*, *20*(1), 381. https://doi.org/10.1186/s12884-020-03075-8

Keedle, H., Peters, L., Schmied, V., Burns, E., Keedle, W., & Dahlen, H. G. (2020b). Women's experiences of planning a vaginal birth after caesarean in different models of maternity care in Australia. *BMC Pregnancy & Childbirth*, *20*(381). https://doi.org/https://doi.org/10.1186/s12884-020-03075-8

Keedle, H., Schmied, V., Burns, E., & Dahlen, H. (2022). From coercion to respectful care: women's interactions with health care providers when planning a VBAC. *BMC Pregnancy & Childbirth*, *22*(1), 70. https://doi.org/10.1186/s12884-022-04407-6

Keedle, H., Schmied, V., Burns, E., & Dahlen, H. G. (2019). A narrative analysis of women's experiences of planning a vaginal birth after caesarean (VBAC) in Australia using critical feminist theory. *BMC Pregnancy & Childbirth*, *19*(1), 142. https://doi.org/10.1186/s12884-019-2297-4

Keedle, H., & Willo, P. (2022). A poetic inquiry of traumatic birth through bearing witness. *Qualitative Inquiry*, *28*(8-9), 938-945. https://doi.org/10.1177/10778004221093424

Kendall-Tackett, K., & Beck, C. T. (2022). Secondary traumatic stress and moral injury in maternity care providers: A narrative and exploratory review. *Frontiers in*

Global Women's Health, 3. https://doi.org/10.3389/fgwh.2022.835811

Kibuka, M., Price, A., Onakpoya, I., Tierney, S., & Clarke, M. (2021). Evaluating the effects of maternal positions in childbirth: An overview of Cochrane Systematic Reviews. *European Journal of Midwifery, 5*(December), 1-14. https://doi.org/10.18332/ejm/142781

Kikuchi, J., Ranjit, A., Jiang, W., Witkop, C., Hamlin, L., & Koehlmoos, T. P. (2020). Early childhood outcomes among infants born by vaginal birth after cesarean and repeat cesarean delivery in the military health system. *Military Medicine.* https://doi.org/10.1093/milmed/usaa536

Kimani, R. W. (2024). Reexamining the use of race in medical algorithms: The maternal health calculator debate. *Frontiers in Public Health, 12.* https://doi.org/10.3389/fpubh.2024.1417429

Kinay, T., Savran Ucok, B., Ramoglu, S., Tapisiz, O. L., Erkaya, S., & Koc, S. (2022). Maternal obesity and intra-abdominal adhesion formation at cesarean delivery. *The Journal of Maternal-Fetal & Neonatal Medicine, 35*(12), 2241-2246. https://doi.org/10.1080/14767058.2020.1783231

Kitzinger, S. (1992). Sheila Kitzinger's letter from England: Birth plans. *Birth, 19*(1), 36-37. https://doi.org/10.1111/j.1523-536x.1992.tb00373.x

Kitzinger, S. (2015). *A passion for birth: My life: Anthropology, family and feminism.* Pinter & Martin Limited.

Kjeldsen, L. L., Dahlen, H. G., & Maimburg, R. D. (2022). Expectations of the upcoming birth - A survey of women's self-efficacy and birth positions. *Sex & Reproductive Health, 34,* 100783. https://doi.org/10.1016/j.srhc.2022.100783

Klagholz, J., & Strunk, A. L. (2009). Overview of the 2009 ACOG survey on professional liability. *ACOG Clinical Review, 14*(6), 1-13.

Kozhimannil, K. B., & Hardeman, R. R. (2016). Coverage for doula services: How state medicaid programs can address concerns about maternity care costs and quality. *Birth, 43*(2), 97-99. https://doi.org/10.1111/birt.12213

Kozhimannil, K. B., Vogelsang, C. A., Hardeman, R. R., & Prasad, S. (2016). Disrupting the pathways of social determinants of health: Doula support during pregnancy and childbirth. *Journal of the American Board of Family Medicine, 29*(3), 308-317. https://doi.org/10.3122/jabfm.2016.03.150300

Kram, J. J. F., Montgomery, M. O., Moreno, A. C. P., Romdenne, T. A., & Forgie, M. M. (2021). Family-centered cesarean delivery: A randomized controlled trial. *American Journal of Obstetrics &Gynecology Maternal Fetal Medicine (MFM), 3*(6), 100472. https://doi.org/10.1016/j.ajogmf.2021.100472

Lakra, P., Patil, B., Siwach, S., Upadhyay, M., Shivani, S., Sangwan, V., & Mahendru, R. (2020). A prospective study of a new prediction model of vaginal birth after cesarean section at a tertiary-care centre. *Journal of Turkish Society of Obstetrics and Gynecology, 17*(4), 278-284. https://doi.org/10.4274/tjod.galenos.2020.82205

Latendresse, G., Murphy, P. A., & Fullerton, J. T. (2005). A description of the management and outcomes of vaginal birth after cesarean birth in the homebirth setting.

Journal of Midwifery & Women's Health, 50(5), 386-391.

Lawrence, A., Lewis, L., Hofmeyr, G. J., & Styles, C. (2013). Maternal positions and mobility during first stage labour. *Cochrane Database of Systematic Reviews,* (10). https://doi.org/10.1002/14651858.CD003934.pub4 Lawton, B., Clarke, M. J., Gibson-Helm, M., & Boyle, J. A. (2021). The lives of women and babies matter: A call for action in Indigenous and First Nations women's health and wellbeing. *International Journal of Gynaecology & Obstetrics, 155*(2), 167-169. https://doi.org/10.1002/ijgo.13929

Leap, N., & Hunter, B. (2016). *Supporting women for labour and birth: A thoughtful guide.* Routledge.

Leinweber, J., Creedy, D. K., Rowe, H., & Gamble, J. (2017). Responses to birth trauma and prevalence of posttraumatic stress among Australian midwives. *Women and Birth, 30*(1), 40-45. https://doi.org/10.1016/j.wombi.2016.06.006

Lubczyńska, A., Garncarczyk, A., & Wcisło Dziadecka, D. (2023). Effectiveness of various methods of manual scar therapy. *Skin Research and Technology, 29*(3). https://doi.org/10.1111/srt.13272

Lundgren, I., Van Limbeek, E., Vehvilainen-Julkunen, K., & Nilsson, C. (2015). Clinicians' views of factors of importance for improving the rate of VBAC (vaginal birth after caesarean section): a qualitative study from countries with high VBAC rates. *BMC Pregnancy & Childbirth, 15*(1). https://doi.org/10.1186/s12884-015-0629-6

Lurie, S., & Glezerman, M. (2003). The history of cesarean technique. *American Journal of Obstetrics and Gynecology, 189*(6), 1803-1806. https://doi.org/10.1016/s0002-9378(03)00856-1

Macedo, D. M., Smithers, L. G., Roberts, R. M., & Jamieson, L. M. (2020). Racism, stress, and sense of personal control among Aboriginal Australian pregnant women. *Australian Psychologist, 55*(4), 336-348. https://doi.org/10.1111/ap.12435

Madaan, M., & Trivedi, S. S. (2006). Intrapartum electronic fetal monitoring vs. intermittent auscultation in postcesarean pregnancies. *International Journal of Gynecology & Obstetrics, 94*(2), 123-125. https://doi.org/10.1016/j.ijgo.2006.03.026

Markou, G. A., Muray, J. M., & Poncelet, C. (2017). Risk factors and symptoms associated with maternal and neonatal complications in women with uterine rupture. A 16 years multicentric experience. *European Journal of Obstetrics,Gynecology, and Reproductive Biology, 217*, 126-130. https://doi.org/10.1016/j.ejogrb.2017.09.001

Matsuzaki, S., Mandelbaum, R. S., Sangara, R. N., McCarthy, L. E., Vestal, N. L., Klar, M., Matsushima, K., Amaya, R., Ouzounian, J. G., & Matsuo, K. (2021). Trends, characteristics, and outcomes of placenta accreta spectrum: a national study in the United States. *American Journal of Obstetrics & Gynecology, 225*(5), 534 e531-534 e538. https://doi.org/10.1016/j.ajog.2021.04.233

McGarry, A., Stenfert Kroese, B., & Cox, R. (2016). How do women with an intellectual disability experience the support of a doula during their pregnancy, childbirth and after the birth of their child? *Journal of Applied Research in Intellectual Disabilities, 29*(1), 21-33. https://doi.org/https://doi.org/10.1111/jar.12155

McLeish, J., & Redshaw, M. (2019). "Being the best person that they can be and the best mum": A qualitative study of community volunteer doula support for disadvantaged mothers before and after birth in England. *BMC Pregnancy & Childbirth*, *19*(1). https://doi.org/10.1186/s12884-018-2170-x

Mercer, B. M., Gilbert, S., Landon, M. B., Spong, C. Y., Leveno, K. J., Rouse, D. J., Varner, M. W., Moawad, A. H., Simhan, H. N., Harper, M., Wapner, R. J., Sorokin, Y., Miodovnik, M., Carpenter, M., Peaceman, A., O'Sullivan, M. J., Sibai, B. M., Langer, O., Thorp, J. M., & Ramin, S. M. (2008). Labor outcomes with increasing number of prior vaginal births after cesarean delivery [Multicenter Study Research Support, N.I.H., Extramural]. *Obstetrics and Gynecology*, *111*(2 Pt 1), 285-291. https://doi.org/10.1097/AOG.0b013e31816102b9

Migliorini, L., Setola, N., Naldi, E., Rompianesi, M. C., Iannuzzi, L., & Cardinali, P. (2023). Exploring the role of birth environment on Italian mothers' emotional experience during childbirth. *International Journal of Environmental Research and Public Health*, *20*(15), 6529. https://doi.org/10.3390/ijerph20156529

Mizzi, R., & Pace Parascandalo, R. (2022). First-time couples' shared experiences of the birth environment. *European Journal of Midwifery*, *6*(October), 1-9. https://doi.org/10.18332/ejm/153946

Modzelewski, J., Jakubiak-Proc, M., Materny, A., Sotniczuk, M., Kajdy, A., & Rabijewski, M. (2019). Safety and success rate of vaginal birth after two cesarean sections: retrospective cohort study. *Ginekologia Polska*, *90*(8), 444-451. https://doi.org/10.5603/GP.2019.0076 Molloy, E., Biggerstaff, D. L., & Sidebotham, P. (2021). A phenomenological exploration of parenting after birth trauma: Mothers' perceptions of the first year. *Women and Birth*, *34*(3), 278-287. https://doi.org/10.1016/j.wombi.2020.03.004

Molyneux, R., Fowler, G., & Slade, P. (2024). The postnatal effects of perineal trauma on maternal psychological and emotional wellbeing: A longitudinal study. *Euroepan Journal of Obstetrics, Gynecology, and Reprod Biology*, *294*, 238-244. https://doi.org/10.1016/j.ejogrb.2024.01.035

Moncrieff, G., Gyte, G. M., Dahlen, H. G., Thomson, G., Singata-Madliki, M., Clegg, A., & Downe, S. (2022). Routine vaginal examinations compared to other methods for assessing progress of labour to improve outcomes for women and babies at term. *Cochrane Database Syst Rev*, *3*(3), CD010088. https://doi.org/10.1002/14651858.CD010088.pub3

Mooney, S. S., Hiscock, R., Clarke, I. D. A., & Craig, S. (2019). Estimating success of vaginal birth after caesarean section in a regional Australian population: Validation of a prediction model. *Australian and New Zealand Journal of Obstetrics and Gynaecology*, *59*(1), 66-70. https://doi.org/10.1111/ajo.12809 Mottl-Santiago, J., Dukhovny, D., Cabral, H., Rodrigues, D., Spencer, L., Valle, E. A., & Feinberg, E. (2023). Effectiveness of an enhanced community doula intervention in a safety net setting: A randomized- controlled trial. *Health Equity*, *7*(1), 466-476. https://doi.org/10.1089/heq.2022.0200

Murray-Davis, B., Grenier, L. N., Plett, R. A., Mattison, C. A., Ahmed, M., Malott, A. M., Cameron, C., Hutton, E. K., & Darling, E. K. (2023). Making space for midwifery in a hospital: exploring the built birth environment of Canada's first alongside midwifery unit. *HERD*, *16*(2), 189-207. https://doi.org/10.1177/19375867221137099

Murshed Alsehimi, O., & Shaban, I. (2021). Exploring maternity healthcare providers' perspectives on maternal upright positions during second stage of labor: A qualitative study. *Egyptian Journal of Health Care*, *12*(4), 233-247.

National Center for Health Statistics. (2025a). *Total cesarean deliveries:*

United States, 2013-2023. March of Dimes. Retrieved 06/01/2025 from https://www.marchofdimes.org/peristats/data?top=8&lev=1&stop=90&reg=99&obj=1&slev=1

National Center for Health Statistics. (2025b). *Vaginal birth after cesarean deliveries*

United States, 2018-2023. March of Dimes. Retrieved 06/01/2025 from https://www.marchofdimes.org/peristats/data?top=8&lev=1&stop=90&reg=99&obj=1&slev=1

NICE. (2019). *Intrapartum care for women with existing medical conditions or obstetric complications and their babies.* https://www.nice.org.uk/guidance/ng121

NMBA. (2018). *Midwife standards for practice.* Nursing and Midwifery Board of Australia. https://www.nursingmidwiferyboard.gov.au/Codes-Guidelines-Statements/Professional-standards/Midwife-standards-for-practice.aspx

NSW Health. (2023). *Integrated trauma-informed care framework: My story, my health, my future.* https://www.health.nsw.gov.au/patients/trauma/Pages/itic-framework.aspx

O'Neill, S. M., Kearney, P. M., Kenny, L. C., Henriksen, T. B., Lutomski, J. E., Greene, R. A., & Khashan, A. S. (2013). Caesarean delivery and subsequent pregnancy interval: A systematic review and meta-analysis. *BMC Pregnancy & Childbirth*, *13*(1), 165. https://doi.org/10.1186/1471-2393-13-165

Oakley, A. (1993). *Essays on women, medicine and health.* DeGruyter.

Office for Health Improvement and Disparities. (2025). *Public Health Profiles.* Retrieved 06/01/2025 from https://fingertips.phe.org.uk/

Oommen, H., Sagedal, L. R., Infanti, J. J., Byrskog, U., Severinsen, M. S., & Lukasse, M. (2024). Multicultural doula support and obstetric and neonatal outcomes: A multi-centre comparative study in Norway. *BMC Pregnancy & Childbirth*, *24*(1). https://doi.org/10.1186/s12884-024-07073-y

Opondo, C., Harrison, S., Sanders, J., Quigley, M. A., & Alderdice, F. (2023). The relationship between perineal trauma and postpartum psychological outcomes: A secondary analysis of a population-based survey. *BMC Pregnancy & Childbirth*, *23*(1). https://doi.org/10.1186/s12884-023-05950-6

Ormsby, S. M., Keedle, H., & Dahlen, H. G. (2025). Women's reflections on induction of labour and birthing interventions and what they would do differently next time: A content analysis. *Midwifery*, *140*, 104201.

Osterman, M. (2020). *Recent trends in vaginal birth after cesarean delivery: United States, 2016–2018* (NCHS Data Brief, no 359. https://www.cdc.gov/nchs/data/databriefs/db359-h.pdfOwens, D. C. (2017). *Medical bondage.* https://doi.org/10.2307/j.ctt1pwt69x

Pairman, S., Tracy, S. K., Dahlen, H. G., & Dixon, L. (2022). Preparation for practice 5e. In: S. Pairman, S. K. Tracy, H. Dahlen, & L.Dixon (Eds.) *Midwifery preparation for practice e-book, 5th Ed.* Elsevier.

Parslow, E., & Rayment-Jones, H. (2024). Birth outcomes for women planning Vaginal Birth after Caesarean (VBAC) in midwifery led settings: A systematic review and meta-analysis. *Midwifery, 139*, 104168. https://doi.org/10.1016/j.midw.2024.104168

Paul, B., Mollmann, C. J., Kielland-Kaisen, U., Schulze, S., Schaarschmidt, W., Bock, N., Bruggmann, D., Louwen, F., Jennewein, L. (2020). Maternal and neonatal outcome after vaginal breech delivery at term after cesarean section - a prospective cohort study of the Frankfurt breech at term cohort (FRABAT). *European Journal of Obstetrics, Gynecology, and Reproductive Biology, 252*, 594-598. https://doi.org/10.1016/j.ejogrb.2020.04.030

Pelak, H., Dahlen, H. G., & Keedle, H. (2023). A content analysis of women's experiences of different models of maternity care: The Birth Experience Study (BESt). *BMC Pregnancy & Childbirth, 23*(1), 864. https://doi.org/10.1186/s12884-023-06130-2

Placek, P. J., & Taffel, S. M. (1988). Vaginal birth after cesarean (VBAC) in the 1980s. *American Journal of Public Health, 78*(5), 512-515.

Pont, S., Austin, K., Ibiebele, I., Torvaldsen, S., Patterson, J., & Ford, J. (2018). Blood transfusion following intended vaginal birth after cesarean versus elective repeat cesarean section in women with a prior primary cesarean: A population-based record linkage study. *Acta Obstetrica et Gynecologica Scandanavica.* https://doi.org/10.1111/aogs.13504

Priddis, H. S., Keedle, H., & Dahlen, H. (2018). The Perfect Storm of Trauma: The experiences of women who have experienced birth trauma and subsequently accessed residential parenting services in Australia. *Women and Birth, 31*(1), 17-24. https://doi.org/https://doi.org/10.1016/j.wombi.2017.06.007

Quattrocchi, P. (2024). *Obstetric violence in the European Union: Situational analysis and policy recommendations.* E. Commission.

Radtke, L., Dukatz, R., Biele, C., Paping, A., Sameez, K., Klapp, C., Henrich, W., & Dückelmann, A. M. (2022). Charité caesarean birth improves birth experience in planned and unplanned caesarean sections while maintaining maternal and neonatal safety: Aprospective cohort study. *Clinical and Experimental Obstetrics & Gynecology, 49*(6), 124. https://doi.org/10.31083/j.ceog4906124

RANZCOG. (2019a). *Birth after previous caesarean section* (best practice statement. https://ranzcog.edu.au/wp-content/uploads/Birth-After-Previous-Caesarean-Section.pdf

RANZCOG. (2019b). *Birth after previous caesarean section..* The Royal Australian and New Zealand College of Obstetricians and Gynaecologists. https://www.ranzcog.edu.au/RANZCOG_SITE/media/RANZCOG-MEDIA/Women%27s%20Health/Statement%20and%20guidelines/Clinical-Obstetrics/Birth-after-previous-Caesarean-Section-(C-Obs-38)-Re-write-July-2015.pdf?ext=.pdf

RANZCOG. (2019c). *Intrapartum fetal surveillance clinical guideline Fourth Ed..* https://

ranzcog.edu.au/wp-content/uploads/Intrapartum-Fetal-Surveillance.pdf

Rastas, L. (2023). Exploring caesarean birth 3: Wound issues and protecting the caesarean wound from surgical wound complications. *The Practising Midwife Australia*, *1*(5), 18-25. https://doi.org/10.55975/poro1042

Reyes Foster, B. M. (2023). "No justice in birth": Maternal vanishing, VBAC, and reconstitutive practice in Central Florida. *American Anthropologist*, *125*(1), 49-62. https://doi.org/10.1111/aman.13796

Roberts, R. G., Deutchman, M., King, V.J., Fryer, G.E., & Miyoshi, T.J. (2007). Changing policies on vaginal birth after cesarean: Impact on access. *Birth*, *34*(4), 316-322.

Rubashkin, N. (2021). *The Mfmu Vbac Success Calculator: Statistical prediction and race in an ethnography of obstetric thinking.* http://ezproxy.uws.edu.au/login?url=https://www.proquest.com/dissertations-theses/mfmu-vbac-success-calculator-statistical/docview/2621260981/se-2?accountid=36155

Rubashkin, N., Asiodu, I. V., Vedam, S., Sufrin, C., Kuppermann, M., & Adams, V. (2024). Automating racism: Is use of the vaginal birth after cesarean calculator associated with inequity in perinatal service delivery? *Journal of Racial and Ethnic Health Disparities.* https://doi.org/10.1007/s40615-024-02233-4

Rucker, M. P., & Rucker, E. M. (1951). A librarian looks at cesarean section. *Bulletin of the History of Medicine*, *25*(2), 132-148.

Saban, A., Shoham-Vardi, I., Yohay, D., & Weintraub, A. Y. (2019). Peritoneal adhesions are an independent risk factor for peri- and post-partum infectious morbidity. *European Journal of Obstetrics & Gynecology and Reproductive Biology*, *241*, 60-65. https://doi.org/10.1016/j.ejogrb.2019.08.001

Sandall, J., Fernandez Turienzo, C., Devane, D., Soltani, H., Gillespie, P., Gates, S., Jones, L. V., Shennan, A. H., & Rayment-Jones, H. (2024). Midwife continuity of care models versus other models of care for childbearing women. *Cochrane Database of Systematic Reviews* (4). https://doi.org/10.1002/14651858.CD004667.pub6

Sandall, J., Tribe, R. M., Avery, L., Mola, G., Visser, G. H. A., Homer, C. S. E., Gibbons, D., Kelly, N. M., Kennedy, H. P., Kidanto, H., Taylor, P., & Temmerman, M. (2018). Short-term and long-term effects of caesarean section on the health of women and children. *The Lancet*, *392*(10155), 1349-1357. https://doi.org/https://doi.org/10.1016/S0140-6736(18)31930-5 Satone, P. D., & Tayade, S. A. (2023). Alternative birthing positions compared to the conventional position in the second stage of labor: A review. *Cureus.* https://doi.org/10.7759/cureus.37943

Schlüter, C., Kraag, G., & Schmidt, J. (2023). Body shaming: An exploratory study on its definition and classification. *International Journal of Bullying Prevention*, *5*(1), 26-37. https://doi.org/10.1007/s42380-021-00109-3

Scholten, N., Strizek, B., Okumu, M.-R., Demirer, I., Kössendrup, J., Haid-Schmallenberg, L., Bäckmann, M., Stöcker, A., Stevens, N., & Volkert, A. (2024). Birthing positions and mother's satisfaction with childbirth: A cross-sectional study on the relevance of self determination. *Archives of Gynecology and Obstetrics.* https://doi.org/10.1007/s00404-024-07770-1

Shinar, S., Agrawal, S., Hasan, H., & Berger, H. (2019). Trial of labor versus elective repeat cesarean delivery in twin pregnancies after a previous cesarean delivery—A systematic review and meta analysis. *Birth, 46*(4), 550-559. https://doi.org/10.1111/birt.12434

Shlafer, R., Davis, L., Hindt, L., & Pendleton, V. (2021). The benefits of doula support for women who are pregnant in prison and their newborns. In *SpringerBriefs in Psychology* (pp. 33-48). Springer International Publishing. https://doi.org/10.1007/978-3-030-67599-8_3

Shorey, S., & Wong, P. Z. E. (2022). Traumatic childbirth experiences of new parents: A meta-synthesis. *Trauma, Violence, & Abuse, 23*(3), 748-763. https://doi.org/10.1177/1524838020977161

Simonovic, D. (2019). *A human rights-based approach to mistreatment and violence against women in reproductive health services with a focus on childbirth and obstetric violence.* https://digitallibrary.un.org/record/3823698?ln=en&v=pdf#files

Sims, J. M. (1886). *The story of my life.* D Appleton & Company.

Small, K. A., Sidebotham, M., Fenwick, J., & Gamble, J. (2020). Intrapartum cardiotocograph monitoring and perinatal outcomes for women at risk: Literature review. *Women and Birth, 33*(5), 411-418. https://doi.org/https://doi.org/10.1016/j.wombi.2019.10.002

Small, K. A., Sidebotham, M., Fenwick, J., & Gamble, J. (2023). The social organisation of decision-making about intrapartum fetal monitoring: An institutional ethnography. *Women and Birth, 36*(3), 281-289. https://doi.org/https://doi.org/10.1016/j.wombi.2022.09.004

Smith-Oka, V. (2022). Cutting women: Unnecessary cesareans as iatrogenesis and obstetric violence. *Social Science & Medicine, 296*, 114734. https://doi.org/10.1016/j.socscimed.2022.114734

Sobczak, A., Taylor, L., Solomon, S., Ho, J., Kemper, S., Phillips, B., Jacobson, K., Castellano, C., Ring, A., Castellano, B., & Jacobs, R. J. (2023). The effect of doulas on maternal and birth outcomes: A scoping review. *Cureus.* https://doi.org/10.7759/cureus.39451

Stamilio, D. M., Defranco, E., Pare, E., Odibo, A., Peipert, J., Allsworth, J., Stevens, E., & Macones, G. (2007). Short interpregnancy interval. *Obstetrics and Gynecology, 110*(5), 1075-1082.

Sun, X., Fan, X., Cong, S., Wang, R., Sha, L., Xie, H., Han, J., Zhu, Z., & Zhang, A. (2023). Psychological birth trauma: A concept analysis. *Frontiers in Psychology, 13*. https://doi.org/10.3389/fpsyg.2022.1065612

Tahseen, S., & Griffiths, M. (2010). Vaginal birth after two caesarean sections (VBAC-2)- A systematic review with meta-analysis of success rate and adverse outcomes of VBAC-2 versus VBAC-1 and repeat (third) caesarean sections. *British Journla of Obstetrics & Gynecology, 117*(1), 5-19. https://doi.org/10.1111/j.1471-0528.2009.02351.x

Takeya, A., Adachi, E., Takahashi, Y., Kondoh, E., Mandai, M., & Nakayama, T. (2020). Trial of labor after cesarean delivery (TOLAC) in Japan: rates and complications. *Archives of Gynecology and Obstetrics, 301*(4), 995-1001. https://doi.org/10.1007/s00404-020-05492-8

Tan, P. C. F., Moran, C. J., & Griffiths, J. D. (2024). Anaesthesia for the maternal-assisted caesarean section. *International Journal of Obstetrics & Anesthesiology, 60,* 104230. https://doi.org/10.1016/j.ijoa.2024.104230

Thisted, D. L. A., Rasmussen, S. C., & Krebs, L. (2022). Outcome of subsequent pregnancies in women with complete uterine rupture: A population based case–control study. *Acta Obstetricia et Gynecologica Scandinavica, 101*(5), 506-513. https://doi.org/10.1111/aogs.14338

Thomas, M.-P., Ammann, G., Brazier, E., Noyes, P., & Maybank, A. (2017). Doula services within a healthy start program: Increasing access for an underserved population. *Maternal and Child Health Journal, 21*(S1), 59-64. https://doi.org/10.1007/s10995-017-2402-0

Thomson, G., Diop, M. Q., Stuijfzand, S., Horsch, A., Lalor, J. G., De Abreu, W., Avignon, V., Baranowska, B., Dikmen-Yildiz, P., El Hage, W., Fontein-Kuipers, Y., Horsch, A., Garthus-Niegel, S., Mesa, E. G., Hadjigeorgiou, E., Healy, M., Inci, F., İsbir, G. G., Jeličić, L., . . . Węgrzynowska, M. (2021). Policy, service, and training provision for women following a traumatic birth: An international knowledge mapping exercise. *BMC Health Services Research, 21*(1). https://doi.org/10.1186/s12913-021-07238-x

Thornton, P. (2018). Limitations of vaginal birth after cesarean success prediction. *Journal of Midwifery & Women's Health, 63*(1), 115-120. https://doi.org/10.1111/jmwh.12724

Thornton, P. D. (2023). VBAC calculator 2.0: Recent evidence. *Birth, 50*(1), 120-126. https://doi.org/10.1111/birt.12705

Thornton, P. D., Liese, K., Adlam, K., Erbe, K., & Mcfarlin, B. L. (2020). Calculators estimating the likelihood of vaginal birth after cesarean: Uses and perceptions. *Journal of Midwifery & Women's Health, 65*(5), 621-626. https://doi.org/10.1111/jmwh.13141

Tinelli, A., Kosmas, I. P., Carugno, J. T., Carp, H., Malvasi, A., Cohen, S. B., Laganà, A. S., Angelini, M., Casadio, P., Chayo, J., Cicinelli, E., Gerli, S., Palacios Jaraquemada, J., Magnarelli, G., Medvediev, M. V., Metello, J., Nappi, L., Okohue, J., Sparic, R., . . . Vimercati, A. (2022). Uterine rupture during pregnancy: The URIDA (uterine rupture international data acquisition) study. *International Journal of Gynecology & Obstetrics, 157*(1), 76-84. https://doi.org/10.1002/ijgo.13810

Todman, D. (2007). A history of caesarean section: From ancient world to the modern era. *Australian and New Zealand Journal of Obstetrics and Gynaecology, 47*(5), 357-361.

Togioka, B., & Tonismae, T. (2021). *Uterine rupture.* StatPearls Publishing. Retrieved 28/02/2021 from https://www.ncbi.nlm.nih.gov/books/NBK559209/

Townsend, B., Fenwick, J., McInnes, R., & Sidebotham, M. (2023). Taking the reins: A grounded theory study of women's experiences of negotiating water immersion for labour and birth after a previous caesarean section. *Women & Birth, 36*(2), e227-e236. https://doi.org/10.1016/j.wombi.2022.07.171

Uebergang, J., Hiscock, R., Hastie, R., Middleton, A., Pritchard, N., Walker, S., Tong, S., & Lindquist, A. (2022). Risk of obstetric anal sphincter injury among women who birth vaginally after a prior caesarean section: A state wide cohort study.

BJOG: An International Journal of Obstetrics & Gynaecology, *129*(8), 1325-1332. https://doi.org/10.1111/1471-0528.17063

Vandenberghe, G., Bloemenkamp, K., Berlage, S., Colmorn, L., Deneux Tharaux, C., Gissler, M., Knight, M., Langhoff Roos, J., Lindqvist, P., & Oberaigner, W. (2019). The International Network of Obstetric Survey Systems study of uterine rupture: a descriptive multi country population based study. *BJOG: An International Journal of Obstetrics & Gynaecology*, *126*(3), 370-381.

Varner, M. W., Thom, E., Spong, C. Y., Landon, M. B., Leveno, K. J., Rouse, D. J., Moawad, A. H., Simhan, H. N., Harper, M., Wapner, R. J., Sorokin, Y., Miodovnik, M., Carpenter, M., Peaceman, A., O'Sullivan, M. J., Sibai, B. M., Langer, O., Thorp, J. M., Ramin, S. M., ... Network, (2007). Trial of labor after one previous cesarean delivery for multifetal gestation. *Obstetrics & Gynecology*, *110*(4), 814-819. https://doi.org/10.1097/01.AOG.0000280586.05350.9e

Vats, H., Saxena, R., Sachdeva, M. P., Walia, G. K., & Gupta, V. (2021). Impact of maternal pre-pregnancy body mass index on maternal, fetal, and neonatal adverse outcomes in the worldwide populations: A systematic review and meta-analysis. *Obesity Research & Clinical Practice*, *15*(6), 536-545. https://doi.org/10.1016/j.orcp.2021.10.005

Vyas, D. A., Jones, D. S., Meadows, A. R., Diouf, K., Nour, N. M., & Schantz-Dunn, J. (2019). Challenging the use of race in the vaginal birth after cesarean section calculator. *Women's Health Issues*, *29*(3), 201-204. https://doi.org/10.1016/j.whi.2019.04.007

Walter, M. H., Abele, H., & Plappert, C. F. (2021). The role of oxytocin and the effect of stress during childbirth: Neurobiological basics and implications for mother and child. *Frontiers in Endocrinology*, *12*. https://doi.org/10.3389/fendo.2021.742236

Wan, S., Yang, M., Pei, J., Zhao, X., Zhou, C., Wu, Y., Sun, Q., Wu, G., & Hua, X. (2022). Pregnancy outcomes and associated factors for uterine rupture: An 8 years population-based retrospective study. *BMC Pregnancy Childbirth*, *22*(1). https://doi.org/10.1186/s12884-022-04415-6

Wasserman, J. B., Abraham, K., Massery, M., Chu, J., Farrow, A., & Marcoux, B. C. (2018). Soft tissue mobilization techniques are effective in treating chronic pain following cesarean section: A multicenter randomized clinical trial. *Journal of Women's Health Physical Therapy*, *42*(3), 111-119. https://doi.org/10.1097/jwh.0000000000000103

Watson, K., Mills, T. A., & Lavender, T. (2022). Experiences and outcomes on the use of telemetry to monitor the fetal heart during labour: Findings from a mixed-methods study. *Women and Birth*, *35*(3), e243-e252. https://doi.org/https://doi.org/10.1016/j.wombi.2021.06.004

Weckend, M., Mccullough, K., Duffield, C., Bayes, S., & Davison, C. (2024). Failure to progress or just normal? A constructivist grounded theory of physiological plateaus during childbirth. *Women and Birth*, *37*(1), 229-239. https://doi.org/10.1016/j.wombi.2023.10.003

WHO. (2009). *WHO recommendations interventions for improving maternal and newborn health.* World Health Organization. https://iris.who.int/bitstream/handle/10665/69509/WHO_MPS_07.05_eng.pdf?sequence=1

WHO. (2018). *WHO recommendations on intrapartum care for a positive childbirth experience.* World Health Organization. https://books.google.com.au/books?id=hHOyDwAAQBAJ

Williamson, K. E. (2021). The iatrogenesis of obstetric racism in Brazil: Beyond the body, beyond the clinic. *Anthropology & Medicine, 28*(2), 172-187. https://doi.org/10.1080/13648470.2021.1932416

Xie, J., Lu, X., & Liu, M. (2024). Clinical analysis of complete uterine rupture during pregnancy. *BMC Pregnancy Childbirth, 24*(1). https://doi.org/10.1186/s12884-024-06394-2

Yuldasheva, A., Omarova, G., Begniyazova, Z., Saduakassova, S., Makhmutova, E., & Meirmanova, A. (2023). Comparison of different cesarean delivery techniques: A systematic review and meta-analysis. *Electronic Journal of General Medicine, 20*(6). https://doi.org/10.29333/ejgm/13590

Zhang, T., & Liu, C. (2016). Comparison between continuing midwifery care and standard maternity care in vaginal birth after cesarean.. *Pakistan Journal of Medical Science, 32*(3), 711-714. https://doi.org/10.12669/pjms.323.9546 Zweifler, J., Garza, A., Hughes, S., Stanich, M. A., Hierholzer, A., & Lau, M. (2006). Vaginal birth after cesarean in California: before and after a change in guidelines. *The Annals of Family Medicine, 4*(3), 228-234.

www.ingramcontent.com/pod-product-compliance
Lightning Source LLC
Chambersburg PA
CBHW072220270326
41930CB00010B/1929